I think this book is a major milestone in the field of qualitative research.... In his demolition of the claims made by a selection of phenomenologists... John Paley has pointed out the emperor's lack of clothing and pushed him into the spotlight for all to see.

Roger Watson, *University of Hull, Editor-in-Chief,*
Journal of Advanced Nursing

Engaging, incisive, forensic.

Alec Grant, *University of Brighton, UK*

The persuasive force and dogged logic of John Paley's argument demands a response. Whether you agree or disagree with him, this book cannot be ignored. It will be required reading for any nurse contemplating undertaking a phenomenological study. Likewise, anyone commenting on phenomenology who does not engage with the arguments Paley advances has not meaningfully engaged with the subject. The influence of this book will ripple through nursing research and education for many years to come.

Martin Lipscomb, *University of Worcester, UK*

Phenomenology as Qualitative Research

Phenomenology originated as a novel way of doing philosophy early in the twentieth century. In the writings of Husserl and Heidegger, regarded as its founders, it was a non-empirical kind of philosophical enquiry. Although this tradition has continued in a variety of forms, 'phenomenology' is now also used to denote an empirical form of qualitative research (PQR), especially in health, psychology and education. However, the methods adopted by researchers in these disciplines have never been subject to detailed critical analysis; nor have the methods advocated by methodological writers who are regularly cited in the research literature.

This book examines these methods closely, offering a detailed analysis of worked-through examples in three influential textbooks by Giorgi, van Manen, and Smith, Flowers and Larkin. Paley argues that the methods described in these texts are radically under-specified, and suggests alternatives to PQR as an approach to qualitative research, particularly the use of interview data in the construction of models designed to explain phenomena rather than merely describe or interpret them. This book also analyses, and aims to develop, the implicit theory of 'meaning' found in PQR writings. The author establishes an account of 'meaning' as an inference marker, and explores the methodological implications of this view.

This book evaluates the methods used in phenomenology-as-qualitative-research, and formulates a more fully theorised alternative. It will appeal to researchers and students in the areas of health, nursing, psychology, education, public health, sociology, anthropology, political science, philosophy and logic.

John Paley was formerly a senior lecturer at the University of Stirling, and is now a visiting fellow at Sheffield Hallam University, UK. He writes on topics related to philosophy and health care, including research methods, evidence, complexity, spirituality, the post-Francis debate about compassion, and nursing ethics.

Routledge Advances in Research Methods

Phenomenology as Qualitative Research

A critical analysis of meaning attribution

John Paley

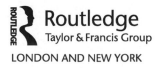

Routledge
Taylor & Francis Group

LONDON AND NEW YORK

First published 2017
by Routledge

2 Park Square, Milton Park, Abingdon, Oxfordshire OX14 4RN
711 Third Avenue, New York, NY 10017

Routledge is an imprint of the Taylor & Francis Group, an informa business

First issued in paperback 2017

British Library Cataloguing-in-Publication Data
A catalogue record for this book is available from the British Library

Library of Congress Cataloging in Publication Data
Names: Paley, John, 1948– , author.
Title: Phenomenology as qualitative research : a critical analysis of meaning attribution / John Paley.
Description: Abingdon, Oxon ; New York, NY : Routledge, 2016. | Includes bibliographical references and index.
Identifiers: LCCN 2016010193| ISBN 9781138652811 (hardback) | ISBN 9781315623979 (ebook)
Subjects: | MESH: Qualitative Research | Ethics, Medical
Classification: LCC R852 | NLM W 20.5 | DDC 610.72–dc23
LC record available at http://lccn.loc.gov/2016010193

ISBN: 978-1-138-65281-1 (hbk)
ISBN: 978-0-8153-5910-4 (pbk)

Typeset in Times New Roman
by Wearset Ltd, Boldon, Tyne and Wear

Contents

Figures

Tables

Acknowledgements

I am grateful to the University of Stirling for granting me a year's sabbatical leave during 2010–11. It was during that year that the book was planned, and several chapters, not all of which are included in the final version, were written.

I am grateful to Sage for permission to quote from *Interpretative Phenomenological Analysis: Theory, Method and Research,* by Jonathan A. Smith, Paul Flowers and Michael Larkin (2009). A number of paragraphs in Chapters 2 and 7 previously appeared in my contribution to *Exploring Evidence-based Practice: Debates and Challenges in Nursing,* edited by Martin Lipscomb for Routledge (2016). Some material in Chapter 7 was originally published in *Nurse Education Today,* Vol. 36 (2015). I am grateful to Taylor and Francis for permission to reuse the former, and to Elsevier and the journal's editor for permission to reuse the latter.

Here is a list of people who, in ways some of them won't recognise, have been supportive and helpful during the last five years: Peter Allmark, Kim Daly, Gail Eva, Lynda Frampton, Fiona Gardiner, Hazel Hill, Trevor Hussey, Richard Lilford, Martin Lipscomb, Olga Petrovskaya, Mark Risjord, Derek Sellman, Paul Snelling. A special word, too, for John Drummond. Critical feedback was provided by Peter, Olga, Gail, Mark, and Paul. In this respect, though, I owe a particular debt to Trevor and Martin, who read just about everything. Probably twice.

I would like to single out Gail for special thanks. I have learned more from her than from anybody else, starting with her time as my PhD student. Discussing anything with her is a rewarding experience, and her thoughts about this project, from its inception, have been invaluable.

Phenomenology is new to Lynda. She likes hearing me talk about it, but she thinks it's a bit weird, and asks challenging, neophyte questions that stop me in my tracks. She has given me a listening ear, a lot of scribbles in the margin, constant laughs, and something that feels very much like home.

I've discussed this stuff with a lot of people over the years, especially at conferences of the International Philosophy of Nursing Society. I am grateful to everybody who listened, questioned, agreed, disagreed, argued, expostulated. I've got to the stage where I have no idea who prompted what thoughts, but I know that many people have left their mark on this book, even if some of them will be aghast to hear me say so. They will be relieved to learn that I don't hold them responsible for its contents.

1 Introduction

The undecided

Let's face it, there are plenty of people who will not be persuaded by this book.

I'm referring to those who do phenomenology. Too much is invested in phenomenological research, too many careers depend on it, and too many papers – hundreds, thousands – have been published, for those who regard themselves as phenomenologists to conclude: 'Maybe he's got a point'. Nor should they. No research programme is dismantled just because there is evidence that contradicts the favoured theory, or arguments that subvert the preferred method. Read Kuhn, read Lakatos.[1] If a research programme can soldier on despite an 'ocean of anomalies' or 'inconsistent foundations' (Lakatos 1978), there is no reason why phenomenologists should pack up and go home merely because their methods are questioned by a single book. Phenomenology will not become an endangered species.

I have a different constituency in mind. The members of this group include the undecided, the waverers, the curious, the provisionally attracted, the secretly baffled, the at-a-loss. They are the ones who are unsure what the alternatives to phenomenology are, and who adopt it not because they are committed to its philosophy – or even have much understanding of it – but because they don't know what else to do. They are the ones who like the general idea, but are wary of the Slough of Philosophical Despond they are expected to wade through. They are the ones who have been nudged along the phenomenological path by an enthusiastic colleague or an insistent supervisor, but who have not yet abandoned themselves to its arcane and hyphenated terminology. A large proportion of this group are postgraduate students.

My main aim is to give this constituency reasons for pausing before they go down the phenomenology route, and to argue that there is an alternative. More than that, it is to provide an indication of what this alternative looks like.

I will do a lot of showing. I will invite readers to look closely at examples of phenomenological analysis in both published studies and methodological texts. This will require a certain amount of patience on the reader's part, and a determination not to let the eye skip and skim over the page, the visual skating act that is often a substitute for reading. Just stop for a moment, I will say, and see what analytical moves the author is making. Do not assume that *her* account of what she is doing can be trusted. Rather: look, then linger, then look again. By slowing the reading down, and taking the author's official description of the analytical process with a pinch of salt, we can see what's really going on.

I'll also ask a lot of questions. The book is stuffed with them. Questions about the passages I invite the reader to examine. Questions about the implications of a particular view. Questions about the apparent inconsistencies in the author's argument. Questions about what has not been said. Questions about how certain terms are used, and what they mean. Questions about why phenomenological writers usually do not explain these terms themselves. My hope is that readers will not merely think about these questions, and have a stab at answering them, but will see that they are of critical importance. Phenomenology is a tradition that discourages certain questions from being asked.[2] One aim of this book is to get those questions into circulation.

So I am trying to persuade the undecided, secretly baffled, at-a-loss constituency; and one of the ways I do that is by inviting them to look closely and ask awkward questions.

PP and PQR

Roughly speaking, there are two types of thing that are called 'phenomenology'. I will refer to them as phenomenology-as-philosophy (PP) and phenomenology-as-qualitative-research (PQR).[3] This book is exclusively about PQR.

Most of the researchers who do PQR assume there is a connection between PQR and PP, and that the methods of PQR are derived, somehow or other, from the work of PP authors such as Heidegger and Husserl. This may or may not be true. Personally, I think it isn't true.[4] But either way, I don't believe the question is relevant to the examination of PQR I undertake in the book. For this reason, I will not talk much about the philosophical comings and goings (at least, not the Husserlian and Heideggerian comings and goings). In particular, I will not suggest that 'phenomenology is both a philosophy and a research method',[5] or that you need to understand PP in order to do PQR.[6]

So 'PQR' refers to a certain form of qualitative research, which might, depending on the affiliations of the writer, be described as 'descriptive phenomenology', 'Husserlian phenomenology', 'Heideggerian phenomenology', 'interpretive phenomenology', 'hermeneutic phenomenology', or some similar label. It usually involves interviewing a small number of people, inviting them to talk about their experience of a particular phenomenon, and analysing the interview transcripts. Often, this analysis culminates in the elucidation of the 'meaning' of the phenomenon concerned. At other times it culminates in a series of themes that characterise the phenomenon, and that are illustrated by excerpts from the data.

An obvious question suggests itself at this point. Given this description of PQR, how precisely does it differ from other types of qualitative method? Other qualitative researchers rely on small samples, ask their respondents to talk about experience, refer to meaning, and identify themes. However, there is presumably something distinctive about PQR, something that differentiates it from these alternatives. What is it? I will call this the 'distinctiveness' question. I suggest a possible answer to it in Chapter 2.

If not the philosophical comings and goings, then ... what? I am interested in how PQR is actually done. So I'll be looking at published examples of PQR, and at the methodological texts cited in the literature. There will be occasional PP asides, but they will usually be restricted to the notes.

Synopsis

There are two main parts of the book. In the first, I review the work of established PQR methodologists: Amedeo Giorgi, Max van Manen, and the trio of Jonathan Smith, Paul Flowers, and Michael Larkin.[7] The focus is mainly on the worked-through examples found in their books. In particular, I am interested in the way in which these authors illuminate, unearth, or elucidate 'the meaning of the phenomenon' in the texts they analyse. It turns out, first, that none of these writers is particularly clear about how this is done; and, second, that the major assumption that they all make about meaning does not appear to be true, even in their own examples. Call this the critical part of the book.

The second part is more constructive. A sizeable chunk of it consists of an analysis of meaning. It is an odd fact that, despite the importance of meaning in PQR studies (and in qualitative methods generally), the concept is rarely discussed in the literature. Questions like the following are not asked: What kind of thing is a meaning? What kind of thing is the 'meaning of a phenomenon'? What kind of thing is the 'meaning of an experience'? How is meaning 'attached' to experience? How is a 'meaning' identified? What practical value does knowing the 'meaning' of something have?

So this book does something PQR authors have not tried to do. It provides an explanation of what meaning *is*.[8]

Having done that, it discusses the methodological implications. This is the positive part of the book. It makes some suggestions about what an alternative approach to interview-based qualitative methods can achieve, and provides an extended example.

I should add, as a matter of reassurance, that I will not be diving into the theoretical differences between the various philosophical heavyweights: Husserl, Heidegger, Gadamer, Merleau-Ponty, Ricœur, and so on. From the point of view of this book, none of that matters. My aim is to encourage the reader to ask questions about the methods described by PQR authors, and to be wary of any answers that are not absolutely clear. The convolutions of phenomenological philosophy can only be a distraction in pursuit of this goal.

In slightly more detail...

Chapter 2 begins with the 'distinctiveness' question. Given that, at first sight, PQR looks like any other type of qualitative research, what is distinctive about it? Is there something that distinguishes PQR from other qualitative genres? My answer is that, in principle, there is. The distinctive feature is an approach to analysis that I will call *meaning attribution*, in which meaning is assigned both to individual units of data, and subsequently to the phenomenon as a whole. Part of the chapter is devoted to explaining this.

However, the situation is complicated by three inconvenient facts. First, many PQR studies lose sight of this distinctive feature of phenomenology, and become what I call 'hybrids': reverting (at least in part) to more generic methods of data analysis. Second, the process of meaning attribution is, for a number of reasons (including hybridisation), largely invisible. We do not know much about how it is carried out in practice because most PQR studies are, at best, sketchy about the details. Third, the concept of meaning attribution gives rise to a series of tricky questions, which the literature does not really answer (or which it answers inconsistently). The chapter briefly considers some of these questions.

There is, however, one aspect of meaning attribution that PQR methodologists seem to be agreed on. Meaning is attributed on the basis of the text, the whole text, and nothing but the text. All three of the methodological works I will be examining insist that an 'analysis attempts to understand the meaning of the description based solely on what is present in the data' (Giorgi); that 'interpretation must be "based on a reading from within the text itself"' (Smith, Flowers and Larkin 2009; from here abbreviated as SFL). In other words, it is illegitimate to make use of 'external' theory.

I call this the *axiom of resident meaning*. Whatever meaning is, it is somehow resident in the data being analysed, or the text being interpreted. It might also be hidden – this is why we need a phenomenologist to find it – but it is nevertheless 'contained' in the data/text.[9] The meaning attributed to a unit of data, or to the phenomenon itself, is not derived from an external source and projected on to the text. Rather, it is distilled from the text itself.

The chapter ends with the question that this discussion poses: *how* exactly is meaning distilled from a text? By what method is it extracted? How is it removed from its hiding place and brought out into the open? Given that PQR researchers hardly ever describe meaning attribution in any detail – although the procedure is obviously pivotal – the answer to this question is by no means obvious.

Chapters 3 and 4 attempt to answer the 'How is it done?' question by examining the way in which the authors of two methods texts (Giorgi, van Manen) do the distilling, describing, illuminating, extracting, elucidating, unearthing, or uncovering.

The structure of these chapters is, perhaps, a bit unusual. Both texts include worked-through examples, intended to illustrate how the recommended method is put into practice. So, in each case, I subject the examples to close scrutiny, considering them on a line-by-line basis in order to determine what can be learned from them. The kind of question I ask is: If Giorgi performs a 'meaning transformation', or if van Manen produces a 'thematic formulation' ... how did they get from *this* to *that*? By what process or procedure did they travel from the *text* to its *meaning*? By what criteria can we evaluate this journey? By what criteria can we say that the proposed move from text-to-meaning is justified (or not)? How do we know if the retrieval of meaning has been done well or poorly?

Chapters 3 and 4 are long, but I hope readers will resist the temptation to skip or skim. Actually, that doesn't just apply to this book. It also applies to the methodological texts I will be examining. Skim those, and you will not notice the glitches. You won't spot the tensions and possible contradictions. For example: if (on one page) van Manen says that experience is pre-reflective and pre-verbal, but if (on another page) he says that experience is 'soaked through with language', you will not notice the apparent discrepancy. As a result, you won't wonder if the two claims can be reconciled, and if van Manen makes any attempt to reconcile them. Nor will you ask yourself whether the contradiction (if it is one) has any methodological consequences and, if so, what they are. In which case, you won't be on the lookout for these potential consequences; and you will not then be able to evaluate their impact.

Chapter 5 is the theoretical centre of the book. The analysis of the methods Giorgi and van Manen use leaves the primary methodological question – 'How is meaning distilled from a text?' – unanswered. It is just not clear, even after working through the examples provided by both authors, how they get from *this* to *that* – from the text to the 'meaning'. This disappointing result is compounded by the fact that neither of them offers any account of what meaning *is*, or how it can be elucidated.

So at this point I present my own account of meaning. I suggest that the words 'means' and 'meaning' are *inference markers*. Their linguistic function is roughly the equivalent of 'therefore'.

It turns out that one consequence of this account is that meaning attribution is impossible in the absence of a background theory. Unlike PQR writers, who say that meaning must not be derived from 'external' theories, my analysis shows that meaning attribution *presupposes* an 'external' theory. In order to test this view, Chapter 6 turns to an example from SFL. The aim is to evaluate their claim that interpretative phenomenological analysis (IPA) should not be based on 'a reading from without', but must be 'based on a reading from within the text itself'. For, if my own account of meaning is correct, a 'reading from within the text' is not possible. So Chapter 6 reviews SFL's example systematically, and shows that their interpretation of the data presupposes a theory that is nowhere to be found in the data itself.

Chapter 7 takes as its premise the idea that 'external theory' is endemic, not only to qualitative analysis, but to the specification of the phenomenon as well, because meaning attribution turns out to be the basis for how a phenomenon is defined. The background theory in phenomenon-definition is always causal, and a properly specified phenomenon always refers to a generalisation based on previous research. For this reason, I distinguish between a *topic* and a *phenomenon*, and suggest that many, perhaps most, PQR studies begin not with a phenomenon but with a topic.

Before developing the idea that theory is intrinsic to qualitative analysis, I attempt to clarify the relation between theories, data and models in scientific enquiry. Taking my cue from recent philosophy of science, I propose that one important function of qualitative research is to use 'some bits of theory and some bits of data' to construct explanatory models.

Most of Chapter 7 provides an extended practical example of how this might be done. Its starting point is a published PQR paper, and it shows how an alternative study, culminating in a model that explains the phenomenon in question, could have been conducted.

A few preliminaries

Three questions will probably occur to the reader, either now or at some point later in the book.

Why these three textbooks?

Because they are the most frequently cited by PQR writers. Other writers are cited in the literature, of course, including Colaizzi (1978), Diekelmann *et al.* (1989), Cohen *et al.* (2000), Dahlberg *et al.* (2001), Creswell (2003), and Lindseth and Norberg (2004). However, Colaizzi's method is a modification of Giorgi's, and the other works are not referenced as often as the three authors examined here.

On what basis did you select published PQR papers for critical attention?

In Chapters 2 and 7, I pick out a small number of published studies for discussion. It is possible that I'll be accused of cherry-picking – selecting weaker studies that are vulnerable to criticism. In fact, I don't think the studies selected for critical attention are unusually weak. I think they are representative of the PQR literature. But I accept that this is a lose-lose situation. I could single out a different permutation of studies, and the same argument could still be made.

As for the criteria of selection, I think there are three. First, the papers are all relatively recent. Second, they are studies that illustrate the critical analysis particularly well because they don't suffer from clutter and complexity (which makes the analysis relatively straightforward). Third, I've avoided papers that are clogged with philosophical discourse. Of course, almost all PQR studies make *some* reference to PP; but most restrict themselves to familiar tropes, and don't attempt to dig any deeper. The selection is from the trope group. I think this is reasonable. It is not as if the philosophically denser studies are noticeably different, methodologically, from the papers that skip more lightly over phenomenological ideas.

Is it worth bothering with the notes?

Many of the notes to Chapters 2 and 7 outline important arguments that would be too much of a detour in the main text. I don't pretend that these notes provide anything more than a sketch. But indicating what the argument would look like is better than providing the argument in full (which would risk losing the main thread) or providing no argument at all. Besides, I use the notes to provide further references, and to indulge myself stylistically (some of them are a bit more colloquial than the main text).

Obviously, it's up to the reader whether they bother with the notes or not. But if they don't, they will miss some of the interest and fun of the book.

Notes

1 Kuhn (1970); Lakatos (1978).
2 It's not just phenomenology, of course. Most traditions do this. In fact, one might almost define a tradition as a way of thinking that suppresses certain questions.
3 Crotty (1996) makes a similar distinction, between 'the phenomenology of the phenomenological movement' and what he calls 'new phenomenology' or 'nursing phenomenology'. These correspond to PP and PQR respectively. Crotty does not think that the 'new phenomenology' is limited to nursing, or that it originated with nursing, since nurses took their PQR methods from education (van Manen) and psychology (Giorgi). But he does suggest that 'a certain understanding of phenomenology has come to the fore in nursing', and that it represents 'a substantial adaptation of mainstream phenomenology'.
4 If anybody wants to check out my previous attempts to explain why, they could consult Paley (1997, 1998, 2005, 2014). Crotty (1996) has comparable arguments. For example: 'This contrast between the laying aside of everyday meaning *[=PP]* and the exploration of everyday meaning *[=PQR]* ... is obvious' (6). Crotty describes PP as critical and objective, while PQR focuses on subjective experience. He has a chapter on 'nursing phenomenology', but is not really interested in PQR as such (though he thinks it has value). He proposes that nurses should develop a style of research that belongs to the PP tradition, and provides an example in his epilogue ('Towards a phenomenology of nursing').
5 As scores of authors do, to the extent that the sentence, 'phenomenology is both a philosophy and a research method', has become almost a mantra. More notable examples include: Morse and Field (1996); Cohen *et al.* (2000); Speziale and Carpenter (2007); Barkway and Kenny (2009); Beck (2009).
6 Some authors make this sort of claim, and send their students off to read *Being and Time*, or some other PP classic, before letting them do any actual research. It is, I would argue, deeply unrealistic to expect nursing postgraduates to have any idea what Heidegger is on about. In fact, it is impossible to understand him without a thorough grounding in philosophy and its history. Even philosophers find him densely difficult and irritatingly opaque. Husserl is indecisive, and can be almost wilfully obscure. There is hardly anybody in philosophy who can tell you, definitively, how the 'phenomenological reduction' is supposed to be carried out (Sparrow 2014). So what chance do postgraduate nurses have?
7 Giorgi (2009), van Manen (1990), Smith *et al.* (2009).
8 I'll state the obvious now, and come back to it later. The 'meaning' of a phenomenon is not the same as lexical meaning. If a PQR writer (Lemay *et al.* 2010) sets out to determine the meaning of fatherhood, she is not referring to the dictionary meaning of the *word* 'fatherhood'. In Chapter 5, I will be asking the question: 'What sort of thing is non-lexical meaning?' What are we talking about when we refer to the meaning of a phenomenon (as opposed to the meaning of a word)?
9 Where the data consists of an interview transcript, it is effectively a text. Clearly, not all data is text, but with PQR studies 'data' and 'text' can be used more or less interchangeably.

References

Barkway, P., and Kenny, D. T. (2009) 'Research for health care practice', in P. Barkway (ed.) *Psychology for Health Professionals*. Chatswood, NSW, Australia: Churchill Livingstone, pp. 104–124.

Beck, C. T. (2009) 'Viewing the rich, diverse landscape of qualitative research', *Perioperative Nursing Clinics*, 4(3), pp. 217–229.

Cohen, M. Z., Kahn, D. L., and Steeves, R. H. (2000) *Hermeneutic Phenomenological Research: A Practical Guide for Nurse Researchers*. Thousand Oaks, CA: Sage.

Colaizzi, P. F. (1978) 'Psychological research as the phenomenologist views it', in R. S. Valle and M. King (eds.) *Existential Phenomenological Alternatives for Psychology*. New York: Oxford University Press, pp. 48–71.

Creswell, J. D. (2003) *Research Design: Qualitative, Quantitative and Mixed Method Approaches*. 2nd edition. Thousand Oaks, CA: Sage.

Crotty, M. (1996) *Phenomenology and Nursing Research*. Melbourne: Churchill Livingstone.

Dahlberg, K., Drew, N., and Nyström, M. (2001) *Reflective Lifeworld Research*. Lund, Sweden: Studentlitteratur.

Diekelmann, N., Allen, D., and Tanner, C. (1989) *The NLN Criteria of Appraisal of Baccalaureate Programs: A Critical Hermeneutic Analysis*. 1st edition. New York: National League for Nursing.

Giorgi, A. (2009) *The Descriptive Phenomenological Method in Psychology: A Modified Husserlian Approach*. Pittsburgh: Duquesne University Press.

Kuhn, T. S. (1970) *The Structure of Scientific Revolutions*. 2nd edition. Chicago: University of Chicago Press.

Lakatos, I. (1978) *The Methodology of Scientific Research Programmes: Philosophical Papers, Volume 1*. Cambridge, UK: Cambridge University Press.

Lemay, C. A., Cashman, S. B., Elfenbein, D. S., and Felice, M. E. (2010) 'A qualitative study of the meaning of fatherhood among young urban fathers', *Public Health Nursing*, 27(3), pp. 221–231.

Lindseth, A., and Norberg, A. (2004) 'A phenomenological hermeneutical method for researching lived experience', *Scandinavian Journal of Caring Studies*, 18, pp. 145–158.

Morse, J. M., and Field, P. A. (1996) *Nursing Research: The Application of Qualitative Approaches:* 2nd edition. London: Chapman & Hall.

Paley, J. (1997) 'Husserl, phenomenology and nursing', *Journal of Advanced Nursing*, 26(1), pp. 187–193.

Paley, J. (1998) 'Misinterpretive phenomenology: Heidegger, ontology and nursing research', *Journal of Advanced Nursing*, 27(4), pp. 817–824.

Paley, J. (2005) 'Phenomenology as rhetoric', *Nursing Inquiry*, 12(2), pp. 106–116.

Paley, J. (2014) 'Heidegger, lived experience and method', *Journal of Advanced Nursing*, 70(7), pp. 1520–1531.

Smith, J. A., Flowers, P., and Larkin, M. (2009) *Interpretative Phenomenological Analysis*. London: Sage.

Sparrow, T. (2014) *The End of Phenomenology: Metaphysics and the New Realism*. Edinburgh: Edinburgh University Press.

Speziale, H. J., and Carpenter, D. R. (2007) *Qualitative Research in Nursing: Advancing the Humanistic Imperative*. Philadelphia: Lippincott Williams & Wilkins.

van Manen, M. (1990) *Researching Lived Experience: Human Science for an Action Sensitive Pedagogy*. Albany, NY: State University of New York Press.

2 Meaning attribution in phenomenology

From a distance, PQR looks like just a standard-issue type of qualitative research, barely distinguishable from other approaches. There is the same emphasis on studying individual experience, the same distrust of quantification, causation, generalisation and truth. Purposive sampling and small-n sample sizes are the norm, the stock-in-trade of data collection is the interview, and PQR studies frequently incorporate a list of themes, just as other genres of qualitative method do.

Bear in mind that I am talking about PQR practice, not the theoretical and philosophical accounts to be found in methods texts. If we consult nurse methodologists, we are told that one distinctive feature of phenomenology is that it is 'both a philosophy and a method' (Cohen 1987; Morse and Field 1995), and that: 'Unfortunately, some phenomenological researchers, especially novices, neglect the philosophical origin of the method' (Holloway and Wheeler 2010: 213). However, it is not always entirely clear what difference this neglect makes, or what novice researchers get wrong as a consequence of neglecting (or possibly misunderstanding) the philosophy in which PQR is grounded.

In this book, however, I am not really interested in 'philosophical origins', or in the connection between PP and PQR. As I have suggested, the primary focus of attention throughout is on what PQR writers *do*, not on what they say.

We should even avoid putting too much faith in the claims researchers make about the distinctiveness of PQR, and why they select it as a method. Many of them say something like: 'Phenomenology was the most appropriate qualitative methodology for this study as it focuses on lived human experience' (Elmir *et al.* 2010: 2533); 'Phenomenological studies ... [seek] in-depth insight into experiences' (Waller and Pattison 2013: 369); 'The approach was selected because the purpose of the study was to understand the meaning of an experience from the perspective of persons who have had that experience' (Phillips and Cohen 2011: 240). The implication is that PQR is especially suited to delivering an 'in-depth insight into experiences', and that the approach was selected precisely for this reason.

However, according to Holloway and Wheeler (2010: 3), qualitative research *in general* 'is a form of social inquiry that focuses on the way people make sense of their experiences'. Similarly, Parahoo (2014: 56) suggests that qualitative research is an umbrella term for approaches 'that seek to understand, by means of exploration, human experience, beliefs, perceptions, motivations, intentions and behaviour'. If this is right, other forms of qualitative research are equally suited to the study of experience. So justifying the selection of PQR because you are seeking insight into experience, or want to understand its meaning, is no justification at all. Other qualitative methods aim to achieve same thing.

It seems unlikely, then, that what makes PQR different from other qualitative approaches will be clearly specified in the work of researchers. In fact, the majority of PQR writers are fuzzy about this, and their attempts to articulate it are rather vague. This may sound odd, as one might assume they would adopt PQR for well-defined methodological reasons. Still, it appears that a lot of PQR is done by people who find it hard to explain what is distinctive about it. And here I mean 'methodologically distinctive', not 'philosophically distinctive'.

In a moment, I will present my own thoughts about what makes PQR distinctive. First, though, I want to make a bit of a detour. I've said that, in practice, PQR is barely distinguishable from other qualitative genres. I think there are some interesting reasons for this, and I would like to explain what they are.

The qualitative research analogous structure

During the past 20–30 years, methodological discussion of qualitative research in health care has been subordinated to the requirements of postgraduate study. The need to maximise publication output has resulted in even master's level research – designed as a display of entry-level competence rather than a contribution to knowledge – appearing routinely in journals; and this has necessitated the legitimation of methods suited to the time-limited, resource-constrained, bums-on-seats MSc enterprise. The process is akin to Darwinian evolution. The academic environment has selected for whatever can be achieved in less than a year, and methodologists have adopted philosophical ideas in order to provide a theoretical justification (Paley 2016).

This evolutionary constraint has imposed certain conditions on postgraduate study. For example, it must be possible to carry out the research in a limited period of time, defined by the deadline for dissertation submission. It must be possible for one person to conduct the study, and for her to be able to do so with very few resources. Given that most students obtained their first degree in nursing or some other health-related field, it must be possible to design the study in the absence of a grounding in relevantly adjacent disciplines, such as psychology or sociology. In view of the vastly increased postgraduate numbers and severe restrictions on time, the intellectual demands must not be too challenging. However, if the study is to be publishable, it must be possible to claim clinical relevance for the research, and to imply that the findings are generalisable.

These conditions are likely to select for designs and methods with the following characteristics:

> *Interview-based.* Other methods, especially participant observation, require a lot of organisation and are difficult to accommodate to fixed timetables and deadlines.

Small samples. The time available to an MSc student permits only a limited number of interviews to be carried out.

Blank slate. Some methodological textbooks recommend that the field of study be approached without any 'preconceived theory'. This limits the amount of reading required, reducing the overall burden on the student.

Study of experience. Focusing on experience means the student does not have to dig too deeply into the theoretical background. A respondent's experience can be described independently of academic theory, so it can be approached without an extensive study of what might otherwise be relevant material.

Description. According to some authors, descriptive studies are the least theoretical types of qualitative research. Consequently, they make fewer demands on students, who do not need to track relevant theory in other disciplines.

Emergent themes. The student burden is further alleviated by an approach to analysis that permits concepts to be generated from the data, rather than from statistics or theoretical sources.

Generalisability. Since it is impossible to justify generalising from small samples on statistical grounds, alternative terms are introduced (for example, transferability), which legitimise generalisation by giving it a different name.

Recipes. Methods which can be reduced to recipes are likely to prove more attractive than those that mean having to start the design process from scratch.

One particularly important recipe determines the formulation of a research aim. It amounts to a kind of pro-forma template (Table 2.1) for a popular type of qualitative study, very often of a PQR kind.

This recipe is admirably suited to postgraduate study because it speeds up the decision-making process. Instead of analysing the literature in order to identify a

Table 2.1 The research on experience template

To	explore/illuminate/identify/elucidate/...*	<description>
the	experience/phenomenon/meaning/...*	<aspect>
of	*insert situation, treatment or condition/...*	<state of affairs>
from the perspective of	patients/nurses/health professionals/...*	<population>
in	*insert location*	<location>

Note
* Select one.

clinical question to which we don't already know the answer – and to justify the claim that an answer to it would be of particular value – the student only has to identify a group of people who have not yet been invited to: 'Tell me about your experience of...'. So the template revises, and considerably simplifies, the concept of a 'gap in the literature'.

I am not, of course, claiming that anybody devised this pro forma, or that students and supervisors ever consciously decide to adopt it. I am claiming that, in the current academic environment, studies that take this form – and that incorporate several of the characteristics outlined above – will be strongly selected for. They will be the default option. Furthermore, they will be a seductive alternative, not just for postgraduate students, but for other qualitative researchers as well. Once the template has evolved, has spawned hundreds of publications, and is legitimated by a series of cheap-and-cheerful philosophical justifications, it becomes available to anybody who is in the business of undertaking qualitative studies.

In evolution, *convergence* occurs when, thanks to the selective pressures of an environment, unrelated species acquire similar biological traits, called *analogous structures*. The wing, for example, evolved separately in birds, bats and insects. In the case of qualitative methods, a number of different 'species' – phenomenology, grounded theory, narrative enquiry, and so on – have all acquired identical traits as a result of adaptation to the postgraduate environment. Though they retain their respective philosophical frameworks, these approaches have converged on the following analogous structure of research practice:

> The retrospective description of experience through small-sample interviewing, both data collection and analysis being carried out in the absence of theoretical preconceptions, with the implicit aim of generalising emergent themes to a population, while explicitly disowning the concept of generalisation.

We might call this the 'qualitative research analogous structure' (or QRAS). It is perhaps the principal reason why, in practice, it is difficult to distinguish phenomenology from other qualitative approaches. Over time, there has been a tendency for all qualitative methods to converge on postgraduate-friendly characteristics. The philosophy, rhetoric, and terminology may diverge, but what people actually do in qualitative research, irrespective of the label they give it, can look pretty much the same.

A brief example of convergent evolution. Glaser and Strauss (1967) show *no* interest in 'experience', and their examples are fieldwork studies based on extensive observation as well as interviews. They do not restrict themselves to description, but propose theoretical explanations linking variables. (For example: the quality of nursing care is a function of the nurse's assessment of the social loss represented by the patient.) Their objective is to generate theory that can subsequently be tested, rather than to perform inductive inferences extrapolating from sample to population. Yet 50 years later, inductive, descriptive, interview-based studies of experience are often classified as 'grounded theory'.[1] Greenfield *et al.* (2012), for example, describe grounded theory as suited to the study of attitudes, motives, feelings, and 'narrative-phenomenological data'.

Three types of conclusion in qualitative studies

Convergent evolution clearly does not entail that different species are alike in every respect. Birds, bats and insects may all have developed wings, but they are still different. So the 'distinctiveness' question still arises: is there anything that distinguishes PQR from other qualitative methods?[2] It's not the focus on experience, it's not the small samples, it's not the in-depth interviews, it's not the emergent themes, and it isn't the philosophical sophistication. So what is it?

In order to answer this question, I must distinguish between three types of conclusion that can be based on – or derived from, or warranted by – a set of qualitative data. Here, 'conclusion' is used as a generic term for any claim that can be supported by data in one of these ways. 'Statement' or 'claim' will do just as well, provided they are understood in this context. The three types can be summarised as follows:

a   *Common themes.* Items of data are assigned to various categories, and the most highly populated categories in a frequency distribution are tabulated as 'common themes'. These are generalisations, limited to the sample, about frequently reported experiences.
b   *Causal hypothesis.* A development of categorisation. Where two categories appear to be associated – that is, constantly linked in the data – a causal hypothesis can be proposed, suggesting that one type of thing typically leads to another type of thing.
c   *Meaning attribution.* Instead of common themes derived from a frequency distribution, or a causal hypothesis based on associated variables, meaning is attributed to individual items of data, and subsequently to the phenomenon as a whole.

I should emphasise, before going any further, that despite the references to generalisation, causation and frequency, I am thinking exclusively about qualitative research, qualitative data, and qualitative analysis. How this is possible should become clear as we proceed.

Common themes

In spite of the hostility to quantification that some qualitative researchers exhibit, it is undeniable that they use quantitative concepts. This point has been made before, especially by Hammersley (1992), who points out that ethnographers routinely use terms such as 'most', 'many', 'frequently', 'sometimes', 'always', and 'regularly'. These may not be precise quantitative concepts, like 'seven' or '23.4 per cent', but they do, nevertheless, refer to amounts or frequencies, and they entail statements that include more precise mathematical expressions. For example, 'most' entails 'more than 50 per cent', and 'sometimes' entails 'on more than zero occasions'.

One of the most frequently used quantitative concepts is 'common themes' or 'commonalities'. These expressions refer, in a non-precise way, to frequency distributions in the data. A 'common theme' is an event, or a state of affairs, or a perception, or an opinion, that turns up in several interview transcripts.[3] In identifying common themes, the qualitative researcher is saying that these events, perceptions, states of affairs (and so on) are reported frequently in situations of the kind being studied. Where the results of the investigation are organised as 'themes', the researcher reports on a frequency distribution. In other words, she makes a generalisation about the sample. This does not, of course, entail a generalisation to the relevant population.

For example, when Kornhaber *et al.* (2015) undertook a PQR study of adult burn survivors, they found that 'the notion of encouragement, inspiration and hope was a clear theme in the transcripts'. In other words, participants often reported finding encouragement, inspiration and hope as a result of talking to other burns survivors. So reports of encouragement as a consequence of this contact had high frequency. This is a sample-restricted generalisation.

In order to identify common themes, there must be categories to which extracts from a transcript can be assigned. The number of extracts assigned to each category can then be counted. Creating categories involves classification. For example, Kornhaber *et al.* (2015) classified encouragement, inspiration, and hope together, taking them to be similar enough to warrant inclusion in the same category. Interestingly, though, they assigned 'reassurance' and 'comfort' to a separate category. This looks a little odd because, *prima facie*, reassurance and comfort appear similar to hope, encouragement and inspiration. However, for reasons that are not explained, they are assigned to a category of their own; and this category consequently becomes a separate theme.

The most likely reason for this classification decision is that 'some participants did not feel comforted or reassured by peer support'. Keeping the two categories separate makes it possible to present *inspiration-hope-encouragement* as having high frequency ('a clear theme'), while acknowledging that *reassurance-comfort* has lower frequency ('some people did not feel comforted/reassured'). The two categories are associated with two themes; but the observed frequency of the items included in each category varies.

Classification into categories permits restricted-to-the-sample generalisations; and that's what 'common themes' are. They are generalisations based on observed frequencies in the sample.[4]

Causal hypothesis

In the terms of quantitative research, common themes are the result of *univariate analysis*. The category is the equivalent of a variable – which has been derived from the data – and 'common' refers to the high frequency with which items assigned to the category are observed in the interview transcripts. Using the same language, a causal hypothesis in qualitative research is an example of *bivariate analysis.*[5]

Typically, a causal hypothesis will link two (sometimes more) variables together. These variables are derived from categories that are observed to co-occur in the data. Simplifying matters a bit, we can say that this hypothesis will usually suggest one of two possibilities:

a   one type of thing generally leads to another type of thing
b   generally speaking, the more of one type of thing there is, the more there will be of another type of thing

Substituting algebraic expressions for 'one type of thing' (x) and 'another type of thing' (y), we get:

a_1 $x \rightarrow y$
b_1 $y = f(x)$

Here, (b_1) says the same as (b), because f (designating a mathematical function) is merely the algebraic equivalent of 'the more ... the more...'.

One of the best known examples of a causal hypothesis is associated with Glaser and Strauss (1967). This hypothesis links two variables: the degree of social loss represented by a dying patient (as assessed by a nurse), and the quality of nursing care afforded to the patient. The hypothesis is of type (b), and says:

The greater the degree of social loss, the higher the quality of care.

The slightly more mathematical way of putting this is to say that: the quality of nursing care is a function of the nurse's assessment of the degree of social loss represented by a dying patient. Mathematically:

$y = f(x)$

where

y = quality of care

x = degree of social loss

f = the mathematical function linking them

The relation between the two variables can even be graphed (Figure 2.1) in a way that provides a rough visual picture of the idea that: the more of x, the more of y.[6]

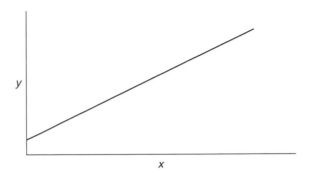

Figure 2.1 Schema of the social loss/quality of care graph.

Like common themes, a causal hypothesis requires a classification scheme by means of which data can be assigned to categories. For example, Glaser and Strauss heard nurses talking about their dying patients in a way that reflected certain aspects of their lives: 'He was so young'; 'He was to have been a doctor'; 'What will the children and her husband do without her?'; 'She had a long and full life' (106). Data items of this sort were collected into a single category labelled 'social loss', and the researchers noticed that in some cases 'social loss' was deemed to be relatively high ('He was so young'), while in others it was deemed to be relatively low ('She had a long and full life'). There were, in other words, degrees of social loss that the patient's death represented (as assessed by the nurses concerned). Further, they noticed that 'patient care tends to vary positively with degree of social loss'. Since 'patient care' is another category, including the range of things a nurse might do for, or on behalf of, the dying patient, there were now two variables that appeared to be associated: 'degree of social loss' and 'quality of patient care'. The more precise version of the causal model proposed by Glaser and Strauss links these two variables:

> The greater the degree of social loss represented by the death of the patient (as assessed by the nurse), the higher the quality of nursing care afforded to that patient.

So the assignment of data items into categories permits, not just the identification of 'common themes' (frequency distributions), but the formulation of a hypothesis causally linking two associated categories. I will say more about causal hypotheses, specifically in the context of model construction, in Chapter 7.

Meaning attribution

Common themes and causal hypotheses depend on categories to which items of data can be assigned: small chunks of data are grouped together under a single heading ('inspiration-hope-encouragement' in the Kornhaber *et al.* example; 'social loss' in the Glaser and Strauss example). Equally, both common themes and causal hypotheses do something that is, in the broadest sense, statistical. In the first case, certain categories are reported to have high frequency; in the second, it is suggested that two variables are associated.

Meaning attributions, on the other hand, do something that is not in any sense statistical, and they are not predicated on categories. Instead of reporting on sample frequencies or suggesting a causal hypothesis, the researcher makes a statement about the *meaning of the phenomenon* being studied. Instead of creating categories into which items of data can be grouped, she elucidates the meaning of individual items. By pooling these item-meanings, she arrives at the meaning of the phenomenon.

Think of it by analogy with a jigsaw, with each piece being an item of data. Depicted on this piece – its meaning, by analogy – is a bit of water, and what might be the stern of a boat. Depicted on this piece, some sky and the edge of a cloud. Depicted on this piece, a fragment of shore. And so on. When all the pieces are fitted together, what emerges is a picture of a sailing regatta on the south coast – analogically, the meaning of the puzzle (=phenomenon) as a whole.

It is evident that the relation between data and conclusion here is different from the corresponding relation in the case of common themes and causal hypotheses. Rather than chunks of data being assigned to categories created by the researcher, every individual item of data now has meaning in its own right. Instead of high-frequency categories being identified as common themes, there is now an overall meaning that can be attributed to the phenomenon under investigation, and that is revealed when all the individual items are assembled. Instead of having to say 'this situation occurs a lot', or 'that view is widely shared', the researcher can now conclude that the meaning of the phenomenon as a whole is ... *X*. For example, the meaning of *persons with chronic pain being approached by health care staff* is: 'an expectation of being encountered as a human with self-worth and dignity' (Hansson *et al.* 2011: 446).

If it is not apparent already, it will become evident later that this account of meaning attribution is not fully transparent, and poses several knotty questions. Before I turn to these questions, however, I would like to suggest an answer to the earlier one: 'What is it that makes PQR different from other forms of qualitative research?'

The distinctiveness of PQR

PQR is, I would argue, differentiated by the fact that it aims at *meaning attribution*, not common themes or causal hypotheses. It attributes meaning to the phenomenon, and achieves this by attributing meaning initially to individual items of data. It does not, at least to begin with, create categories, and it does not engage in anything even broadly statistical.

Causal hypotheses, as my example implies, are typical of grounded theory, or those forms of grounded theory that are more closely derived from Glaser and

Strauss (1967), rather than, for example, Charmaz (2014). However, they are not exclusive to grounded theory, as they often appear in other approaches to qualitative research (for example: Pawson and Tilley 1997; Silverman 2000; Maxwell 2012).

In practice, sample frequencies are a generic option, the default approach to the analysis of data derived from interviews about people's experience. Categories are created, common themes are identified, and the findings section of the research report is devoted to a description of these themes, usually illustrated by extracts from the transcripts. Probably a majority of qualitative studies in nursing – irrespective of the methodological or philosophical label attached to them – take this form.

In summary, PQR is that form of qualitative research that focuses on experience, and that engages in meaning attribution. This concept determines both the primary aim of a PQR study – to elucidate the meaning of a phenomenon – and the primary method of achieving that aim: the attribution of meaning to individual units of data.

Essence

Sometimes PQR authors and methodologists talk about the 'essence' of a phenomenon in addition to (or instead of) the 'meaning'. For some writers, this concept has particular importance. Van Manen (1990), for example, states that 'phenomenological research is the study of essences'. The problem, however, is that he (like many other writers) never explains what he means by 'essence', and he runs it together with other ideas. In particular, he riffs through different permutations of *essence, meaning, nature, essential structure,* and *phenomenon,* without ever clarifying the relation between these terms. Consider what he says about the ultimate objective of phenomenological studies. Phenomenology aims to:

understand the lived structures of meaning (4)

understand the nature or meaning of our everyday experiences (9)

uncover the internal meaning structures of lived experience (10)

study essences (10)

ask 'What is the nature or essence of the experience of…?' (10)

ask what is it that constitutes the nature of this lived experience (32)

ask, what is the nature of the phenomenon as meaningfully experienced (40)

grasp the essential meaning of something (77)

determine the experiential structures that make up that experience (79)

The impression this creates is that van Manen is indifferent to the possible distinctions implied by, for example, 'essence', 'meaning' and 'nature'.[7] These apparently diverse concepts are, from his point of view, nothing more than variations on a theme. The lived structure of meaning, the internal meaning structure of lived experience, the nature or meaning of experience, the nature or essence of experience, the nature of the phenomenon, the essential meaning, and experiential structures ... all appear to be ways of referring to the same thing.

Van Manen offers no theory here. Instead, he gives us an array of effectively synonymous expressions, whose purpose is to persuade us that the phenomenologist is in a position to tell us something *profound* about a phenomenon, which we might not otherwise have noticed. Precisely what we call that profound something-or-other does not seem to be relevant.

Following van Manen's lead, the PQR research literature does not make a distinction between 'meaning' and 'essence'. For example, Monaro *et al.* (2014) conclude that the *essence* of the early haemodialysis experience is a 'lost life'. Herlin and Wann-Hansson (2010) suggest that the *meaning* of haemodialysis is 'a total lack of freedom'. Moran *et al.* (2010) conclude that the *overarching pattern* of haemodialysis is 'waiting for a kidney transplant'. None of these authors says anything about whether an 'essence', a 'meaning', and an 'overarching pattern' are the same or different. What they all take themselves to be doing is identifying a critical, or central, or perhaps defining, attribute of the experience concerned. It is this critical/central/defining attribute that appears to be what PQR writers are aiming at, and the label that gets attached to it – essence, nature, meaning, structure, pattern – doesn't really matter.

In PQR discourse, then, 'meaning', 'essence', 'nature', 'essential structure', and 'overarching pattern' are all labels for a kind of précis: that is, a summary statement that expresses something profound and non-obvious about the experience concerned. It is this précis, together with meaning attribution, that is the alternative to common themes and causal hypotheses, and which is the distinguishing mark of PQR.

An immediate qualification: hybrids

This account of the distinctive features of PQR is based on what the textbooks say, rather than research studies. Van Manen (1990) argues that human science, which he identifies with phenomenology, 'aims at explicating the meaning of human phenomena'. His method involves developing 'thematic formulations' for each unit of data, where 'theme' is understood as 'the experience of focus, of meaning, of point'; and he notes that the 'theme is my tool for getting at the meaning of the experience', though he also observes that 'no thematic formulation can completely unlock the deep meaning'. Similarly, Smith *et al.* (2009) argue that IPA research questions need 'to be directed towards "meaning"' rather than causation; while Giorgi's (2009) method is the definition of 'meaning units' and the 'meaning transformations' that are performed on them.

However, things do not look so clear cut when we consider published research. The principal reason for this is the qualitative research analogous structure. The convergence on QRAS has encouraged hybrids that adopt the language of meaning attribution, but in practice combine it with a 'common themes' or 'causal hypothesis' strategy. Typically, the discrepancy between 'meaning attribution' discourse and the 'common themes' or 'causal hypothesis' organisation of findings is not acknowledged.

A few examples. Glenn *et al.* (2014) base their hermeneutic phenomenological approach on Creswell's (2003) 'steps for interpreting qualitative data'. The procedure involved colour-coded words and phrases, which were subsequently placed into 26 categories. These categories were then amalgamated into five themes. So far, this appears to be a 'common themes' study, something confirmed by references to 'five major areas', with documentation being 'a major theme'. However, once the themes were established, the 'transcripts were reviewed to determine which statements best captured the fundamental *meanings* of these themes' (Glenn *et al.* 2014: 2025); and 'the *essence* of the phenomena was developed on further reflection on these themes' (2026).

The 'essence' statement, given a section to itself, is worth quoting:

> Caring Nurse Practice, defined as nurturing care, advocacy and education in the nurse-patient relationship, is in and of itself complex. During the second stage of labour, pushing that is allowed to occur naturally, contributory interactions with the healthcare team and participation in perinatal safety initiatives and Relationship-Based care models reduce complexity and may improve outcomes. Complexity is increased in response to disruptive interactions with the healthcare team along documentation demands of a non-intuitive electronic health record, which may result in suboptimal outcomes.
>
> (2026–2027)

The authors do not spell out precisely what this is the essence *of*, but I assume that they have 'caring nursing practice' in mind. Two basic claims are made here, after the opening sentence. First, various factors (natural pushing, contributory interactions, and so on) reduce complexity and may improve outcomes. Second, disruptive interactions increase complexity, and may result in suboptimal outcomes.

These are clearly causal hypotheses, with two cause/effect links rather than one. Several factors reduce complexity; and reduced complexity improves outcomes. Similarly, two factors in particular increase complexity; and increased complexity results in suboptimal outcomes. We can represent this as follows (where 'F' = factor, 'C' = complexity and 'O' = outcomes):

$$F_1 + F_2 + F_3 + F_4 \rightarrow C^{decreased} \tag{1}$$
$$C^{decreased} \rightarrow O^{improved}$$

$$F_5 + F_6 \rightarrow C^{increased} \tag{2}$$
$$C^{increased} \rightarrow O^{suboptimal}$$

However, this is not the only way the causal hypotheses can be represented. One factor appears in both the first and second claims: interactions with the healthcare team. If these are 'contributory', complexity is decreased (and outcomes improve). If they are 'disruptive', complexity is increased (and outcomes are suboptimal). The link between interactions and outcomes can be represented as a graph (Figure 2.2), where:

y=outcomes, varying from good (g) to poor (p)

x=interactions, varying from maximally contributory (+) to maximally disruptive (−)

By the same token, this hypothesis can be represented as a mathematical equation:

$$y = f(x)$$

Where:

f=the mathematical function linking interactions and outcomes

The graph and equation represent only one of the causal links entailed by the two hypotheses. Clearly, the causal situation is more complicated than this one equation suggests, given that other factors are implicated. But I am using this example to demonstrate that the 'essence statement' is in fact a causal claim, proposing that various factors lead to improved or suboptimal outcomes. If it is true (in this case) that y=f (x), there would clearly be an argument for making interactions with the healthcare team more 'contributory' and less 'disruptive'.[8]

So, although it is described as an 'essence statement', the quoted passage proposes a causal hypothesis about the effects of caring nursing practice on patient outcomes. Of course, it can't be both an 'essence' statement *and* a causal

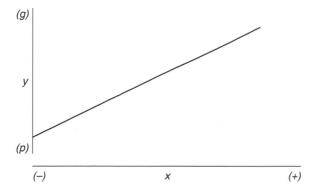

Figure 2.2 Schema of the interactions/outcomes graph.

hypothesis. We must be able to distinguish between the essence of X (smoking, for example) and the effects of X. The *essence* of smoking (inhaling tobacco smoke) is one thing, the *effect* of smoking (cancer) is another. Confusing the two would make studies of the causal consequences of smoking redundant. Similarly, the essence of 'caring nursing practice' cannot include its (alleged) effectiveness.

It is no accident, of course, that Glenn *et al.* (2014) is based on self-reports by nurses who provide intrapartum care. Indeed, the nurses were asked to describe the 'effects of healthcare environment, system, or personnel'. So it cannot be surprising that contributory interactions and relationship-based care models were reported as being conducive to good outcomes. This is precisely what one would expect nurses to say. Equally, it is no surprise that nurses dislike non-intuitive electronic health records and 'disruptive interactions', and claimed that these were conducive to suboptimal outcomes. Of course, they *might* be correct. But the fact that 13 nurses from a single hospital *believe* that 'non-intuitive electronic health records' lead to suboptimal patient outcomes does not constitute evidence that they actually do. In legal terms, this is not much better than hearsay; and it is extremely likely that self-serving bias would incline nurses to present their own contribution to health care in a positive light.

In another self-report study, Atsalos *et al.* (2014), the effectiveness of nurse consultants is presupposed in the very definition of the phenomenon to be studied. This example of 'hermeneutic phenomenology' set out to develop new insights into 'the phenomenon of clinical nurse/midwifery consultant clinical effectiveness in a tertiary referral hospital'. This is a study that could have asked a causal question: do certain interventions (*x, y* or *z*) of clinical nurse consultants have good outcomes for patients? Instead, it asks nurse consultants to talk about their experiences. The authors just assume that the consultants *are* clinically effective.

The findings, unsurprisingly, are relentlessly positive. The 15 consultants (from one hospital) 'focus primarily on the facilitation of the patient experience and the optimisation of care'. They frequently take 'responsibility for ensuring effective continuity of care'. They all have the 'ability to develop a trusting relationship with patients'. They can 'anticipate the unexpected', 'anticipate what others may not have foreseen', and are 'unrestricted by preconceived expectations'. They can 'supplant the narrow focus of routine with a broader perspective', 'question the obvious', and 'prevent otherwise unforeseen adverse outcomes'. The consultants 'display a resolute determination to move public health care forward', and 'are accustomed to acting decisively and effectively in difficult situations'. When faced with obstacles, they 'dig deeply' into their 'rich tapestry of experience', simultaneously 'tapping into every area they can'. They attempt to 'break through restrictions placed on them by entrenched systems and processes'. They 'take leading roles in the redesign of existing clinical services' and the initiation of 'new multi-disciplinary projects', managing to overcome the associated problems. Most of them are involved in regional or national committees, 'generally in their own time and at their own expense' (Atsalos *et al.* 2014: 2878–2880).[9]

The researchers know all this, let us recall, because the consultants told them it was so.

This is mind-boggling. The consultants are paragons of clinical competence, with a breathtaking range of skills and achievements. The only circumstances in which they are less than exceptional is when they face insuperable obstacles, all of which are created by other people. Of course, none of this is surprising. The researchers just assume that the consultants are effective, and ask them to talk about how they do it. The consultants are apparently only too willing to oblige.

The researchers record these stories, identify the most frequently reported abilities and accomplishments, and present them as a series of 'new insights into the phenomenon'. Despite reference to the 'extensive interpretive hermeneutic analysis', 'ontological understandings', 'lived experience', the 'hermeneutic circle', and 'uncovered meanings', the findings resolve into the familiar 'frequency' pattern (Atsalos *et al.* 2014: 2874). The study is at best a hybrid. Strip out the Heideggerian vocabulary, and it is simply another example of 'common themes' qualitative research.

An even more transparent example of a hybrid is Ernersson *et al.* (2010). In this study, 18 participants (all young and healthy) were given what even the authors call an 'intervention', and were subsequently interviewed in order to determine its effects on them. The intervention consisted of a sedentary lifestyle and increased food intake (described as 'obesity provoking behaviour') over a four-week period. This is, by any estimation, a quasi-experimental study, with the effects of the intervention being gauged through a qualitative interview rather than by structured outcome measures.

However, for reasons that are not fully explained, the authors force the study into a 'meaning attribution' framework, adopting Giorgi's (1985, 1997) method. They 'determine meaning units', 'transform' them into the 'language of nursing', and then synthesise them into 'essential meaningful patterns'. 'Reduction was performed', and in this phase 'the main essence and five structures emerged' (Ernersson *et al.* 2010: 567).

But it is quite obvious, reading the results section, that the 'main essence of the phenomenon' refers to the '*most frequently reported effects* of the intervention'. Here is the authors' summary of the findings: 'The main essence of the phenomenon, adopting an obesity provoking behaviour was lack of energy'. This included feelings of tiredness, sleep problems, breathlessness, reduced self-esteem and a deleterious impact on the participants' sex life (ibid.: 567).

These findings are predictable, but that is not the key issue. The main point is that this is an intervention study, in which an attempt has been made to evaluate the effects of more calories and less exercise on healthy individuals. However, the findings are organised as a set of frequencies. The authors say that 'the *most common* experience was a pronounced lack of energy'. In addition to these common themes, there is a causal claim, based on self-report: the intervention had the impact reported by the participants.

The study is, in fact, something of a mishmash. Frequently reported experiences are tabulated, a causal hypothesis is implied … and the whole is swaddled in phenomenological terminology. 'Meaning units' are identified, 'meaning transformations' are carried out, and the outcomes are described as 'essences'. There is obviously a prior commitment to phenomenology as a method. However, the QRAS has exerted its magnetic pull, and the study has ended up as a methodological mongrel.

This, as I have said, is not an uncommon situation. The ideological commitment to phenomenology is strong, but the environmental factors selecting for QRAS are equally powerful, and the result is often something that falls between two stools. In extreme cases, an ostensibly PQR study is just a 'common themes' investigation, with the familiar repertoire of phenomenological references providing no more than terminological garnish.

Meaning attribution in practice

The fact that studies like those discussed in the previous section are hybrids does not necessarily mean that they fail to include meaning attributions at some point in the analytical process. However, given the abbreviated length of most journal articles, PQR studies do not usually include detailed accounts of data analysis, so it is often impossible to work out precisely what procedures have been followed.

For example, Ødbehr *et al.* (2015) adopted van Manen's 'hermeneutical phenomenological' approach because they 'sought a deeper understanding of the meaning of the nurses' experiences'. Here is their summary of the analytical process (362):

> We attempted to let the text 'speak' to us and we were influenced by the text in a non-cognitive way, searching for both the apparent and deeper meaning in the text. For example, a section of text stated that the nurses felt *embarrassed* when singing religious songs.... In the light of the text in its entirety, the 'deeper meaning' of the text could be that faith and religiosity are a personal matter in the Norwegian society that should not be expressed openly. The text was divided into meaningful units and condensed; throughout we emphasized that the meaning of the text was preserved. Our assumptions and pre-understandings were explicated by our openness and reflection. During the reading of the interview text, we reflected on the essential topics to uncover the significance of a certain experience and commonalities between the experiences. We also reflected on the parts of the text that seemed obscure by repeatedly questioning the text. During this work, we identified themes and clusters of themes that constituted sub-themes and, subsequently, main themes.

Those already committed to PQR, and to its supposed philosophical background, will not find anything here to puzzle them. The passage includes some familiar phenomenological tropes, which readers who belong to the PQR community will assume they understand. To the outsider, however, expressions such as 'deeper meaning', 'the meaning of the text', 'reflection', 'questioning the text', 'meaningful units' 'essential topics', and 'pre-understandings' are exasperatingly non-transparent. Although they appear to present a methodological narrative, they are frustratingly uninformative, and tell the uninitiated nothing about what the researchers actually *did*.

To see this, consider a list of questions that the passage provokes, and which the authors signally fail to answer:

- What does it mean to say that the text 'speaks' to the researcher?
- How does the researcher go about letting the text do this?
- What is the 'non-cognitive' influence that the text exerts, and how is it exerted?
- What difference does the 'text in its entirety' make?
- In what way does a 'deeper meaning' differ from the 'apparent meaning'?
- Why is this an important distinction?
- How does the researcher know when she has identified the deeper meaning?
- Why is faith-as-a-personal-matter a deeper meaning, and in comparison to what?
- What are meaningful units, and how are they identified?
- In what sense are meaningful units condensed?
- What kind of activity is 'preserving the meaning of the text'?
- How was the meaning of the text preserved, and why was this necessary?
- What are pre-understandings?
- In what sense are assumptions and pre-understandings 'explicated'?
- What kind of reflection makes it possible to explicate one's pre-understandings?
- How is this reflection carried out?
- How does the researcher know that she is carrying out this reflection correctly?
- What are the 'essential topics'?
- How are the essential topics identified?
- In what sense does an experience have 'significance'?
- How is that significance uncovered?
- What kind of activity is 'questioning the text'?
- How is this questioning carried out?
- What answers, in this case, did the text give?
- How did the researcher recognise these answers?

Unless these questions are answered, we literally do not know how the analysis was undertaken. Again, I suspect that those signed up to PQR will be inclined to treat my scepticism impatiently. *They* know what is meant; *they* can decode metaphors such as the 'text speaking to the researcher', 'questioning the text', 'deeper meaning', and 'uncovering significance'. They understand how a researcher identifies essential topics, meaningful units, themes and pre-understandings. They recognise these things because they've been there, done that, got the paper published. They are unimpressed by somebody asking questions they already know the answers to.

Personally, I think this is a form of self-deception. For example, take the quest for a 'deeper meaning'. If the researcher does not specify criteria for what *counts* as a 'deeper meaning'; if she fails to explain how she *identifies* the 'deeper meaning'; if she does not say why the 'deeper meaning' is *important* and what we're supposed to do with it; if she does not (in this particular case) spell out the relation between the 'deeper meaning' of the text and a *sociological theory* of faith and religiosity in Norway (Furseth 2005; Repstad 2009; Zuckerman 2007); then why should the reader looking for solid evidence take any notice of her? It is all very well claiming to understand the terminology, and nodding sagely when others use it; but unless it can be explained clearly to those who stand outside the inner circle of phenomenological researchers, then studies that rest on PQR methods are going to have very little traction. In addition to which, there is always the suspicion that if a writer cannot explain her methods to someone else, there is a distinct possibility that she does not really understand them herself.

There is a sense in which PQR has inherited an endemic vagueness about method from phenomenology-as-philosophy. As Sparrow (2014) points out, Husserl was never satisfied with his account of method in phenomenology, and left his followers with no clear statement of how to conduct a phenomenological investigation.

> If the method of phenomenology is uncertain, it is difficult to see how its results could be reliable.... A method is supposed to rein in spurious conjecture and speculative impulses, not send out search parties in every possible direction.
>
> (3–4, 5)

Having recourse to 'deeper meaning', 'reflection', and 'letting the text speak' is not far removed from 'sending out a search party'; and the problem associated with depending on such vague abstractions is that it provides no means of distinguishing between good evidence and 'spurious conjecture'. Without the 'reining in' function of an explicit method, references to 'the deeper meaning', or 'letting the text speak', can become camouflage for 'finding in the text what I want to find' – not as a deliberate act of deception, but as a result of the researcher first deceiving herself.[10]

The Ødbehr *et al.* (2015) paper is by no means unusual in relegating critical methodological details to an off-stage role, restricting the on-stage, public performance to resonant but uninformative gestures. The idea of meaning, and the activities of interpreting for meaning, revealing meaning, disclosing meaning, understanding meaning, formulating meaning, uncovering meaning, clarifying meaning, transforming meaning, going beyond the literal meaning, and identifying meaning units, are constantly referred to, but never illustrated, explained, elaborated, or examined (for example: Lindy and Schaefer 2010; Burhans and Alligood 2010; Scheckel *et al.* 2010; Phillips and Cohen 2011; Monaro *et al.*

2014; Torresan *et al.* 2015). I accept that this is sometimes because of limited space; but the fact remains that we know almost nothing about the basis for meaning attribution in PQR. It is, for all practical purposes, invisible.

Questions about meaning attribution

We have arrived, then, at a somewhat paradoxical conclusion. On the one hand, I have suggested that meaning attribution is the only feature of PQR that can distinguish it from other genres of qualitative research. On the other, we do not have much idea how, in practice, meaning attribution is carried out because published studies provide little more than sketches. In any case, thanks to the gravitational pull of QRAS, studies that are ostensibly PQR often turn out to be hybrids, grafting the discourse of meaning attribution on to common themes and/ or causal hypotheses.

In the middle chapters of this book, I will scrutinise examples of meaning attribution in the work of PQR methodologists in order to get a clearer answer to the question 'How is it done?'. First, however, I want to draw attention to a number of other questions that the idea of meaning attribution seems to prompt.

The meaning of what?

PQR authors tend to be somewhat imprecise about what it is they attribute meaning *to*.[11] Consider SFL (Smith *et al.* 2009), for example. They offer various descriptions of the object of phenomenological enquiry – what it is that interpretative phenomenological analysis (IPA) 'explores' or 'is concerned with'. These descriptions vary a great deal. At different points in their book, we find:

the thing itself	(186)
the thing itself as it appears to show itself	(24)
how something is	(30)
how a phenomenon appears	(28)
the phenomenon ready to shine forth	(35)
lived experience	(11)
experience on its own terms	(1)
what the experience of being human is like	(11)
people's meaning-making activities	(18)
the content of consciousness	(16)

It is by no means obvious that these are identical. For example, 'the content of consciousness' appears, at first sight, be something significantly different from 'the thing itself'. Similarly, it is not self-evident that 'how something is' can be identified with 'meaning-making activities'. Nor is it obvious that 'lived experience' is the same as 'the phenomenon ready to shine forth'. Further, 'the thing itself' could be one thing, while 'the thing itself as it appears to show itself' could be another.

No doubt it would be possible to tell a story explaining why each of these descriptions refers to the same thing, or at any rate a story explaining how they are related to each other. Unfortunately, SFL do neither. Instead, they leave it to the reader to devise a coherent framework in which they can all be fitted neatly together. This is not untypical of PQR authors.

To the uninitiated, it seems obvious that there are different objects of study. The *thunderstorm itself* is one thing; the *experience of thunderstorms* is another; the individual or cultural *meaning attached to thunderstorms* is a third. That's three disciplines already – meteorology, psychology and anthropology – with the 'contents of consciousness' and the 'phenomenon ready to shine forth' still unaccounted for. On what grounds, then, do PQR writers ignore these distinctions? Do they believe that the *thing itself*, the *experience*, and the *contents of consciousness* are all the same thing, to be studied in the same way? If so, why?

Surprisingly, despite the pivotal nature of these concepts in PQR studies, they are never explained. There are, as far as I am aware, no attempts to say exactly what a 'phenomenon' is,[12] or how phenomena can be identified; no discussion of the different senses of 'experience';[13] no analysis of 'essence'; no theory of 'meaning'. The PQR literature treats these concepts as if they were transparent, and in no need of analysis or explanation. The conceptual foundations of PQR, that is to say, have never been examined.

What kind of meaning?

In what sense does a phenomenon have meaning? It is presumably not the lexical sense.[14] For example, if someone refers to the meaning of the phenomenon *being 30–45 years of age and depending on haemodialysis treatment* (Herlin and Wann-Hansson 2010), they are presumably not referring to the dictionary meaning of the words in italics. So what kind of 'meaning' are they referring to?

Moreover, when Herlin and Wann-Hansson say that the meaning of this phenomenon is 'a total lack of freedom', what are they intending to convey, and what significance does this claim have? Wouldn't the meaning of the phenomenon *being in prison* be a 'total lack of freedom' too? In which case, what is the relation between the meaning of *being 30–45 years of age and depending on haemodialysis treatment* and the meaning of *being in prison*? Can the phenomenon *being 30–45 years of age and depending on haemodialysis treatment* and the phenomenon *being in prison* both have the same meaning? If so, how can this be explained? What does 'meaning' designate in this context?

Authors refer variously to primary meaning, secondary meaning, deeper meaning, subjective meaning, literal meaning, essential meaning, perceived meaning, core meaning and lived meaning[15] (for example: Burhans and Alligood

2010; Hansson *et al.* 2011; Tavakol *et al.* 2012; Cheng *et al.* 2013; Monaro *et al.* 2014; Ødbehr *et al.* 2015; Torresan *et al.* 2015). What distinctions are implied by these expressions? Do some of them refer to the same thing? Is 'secondary meaning' the same as 'deeper meaning'? Is either of them the same as 'essential meaning', 'core meaning', or 'exact meaning'? Is 'lived meaning' a synonym of 'subjective meaning', or 'perceived meaning'? Is 'primary meaning' the same as 'literal meaning'? Or is the latter equivalent to dictionary meaning, while 'primary meaning' and 'secondary meaning' refer to ... something else? What's remarkable is that all these expressions are used casually, as if what they mean were obvious, and as if the relations between them were self-evident. None of these authors indicates exactly what they have in mind, or explains the significance of the distinctions they draw.

Intrinsic or attached?

Some PQR authors talk as if meaning is *intrinsic* to the phenomenon concerned, others talk of meaning being *attached* to the phenomenon (or experience) by the participant. Examples of the first type: Thurang *et al.* (2010); Herlin and Wann-Hansson (2010); Galvin and Timmins (2010). Examples of the second type: Crotser and Dickerson (2010); Vuori and Åstedt-Kurki (2013); Wilson (2014). Many other papers appear to be ambiguous in this respect (Thorkildsen and Råholm 2010; Kouwenhoven *et al.* 2011; Little 2012).

The difference between intrinsic meaning and attached meaning looks as if it should be a sharp one. On the one hand, there is the idea that a phenomenon has a certain meaning intrinsically, irrespective of who experiences it. On the other, there is the idea that people affix their own meaning to a phenomenon, and that this is specific to the individual concerned.

However, the distinction is perhaps not as clear-cut as it initially seems. It might be suggested that, by integrating (in some sense) the attached meanings of individual respondents, the intrinsic meaning of the phenomenon can be identified. And the most obvious candidate for the relevant type of 'integrating' is an analysis that picks out meanings that were attached by *all* the respondents, on the understanding that these 'common meanings' must be the intrinsic ones (must, in other words, be attributable to the phenomenon itself).

This suggestion prompts a couple of tricky questions. First, what justifies the assumption that meanings attached to a phenomenon by every member of a small group of respondents (who are often confined to a single area or institution) must be those which belong to the phenomenon intrinsically? How do we know that the meanings common to that group are not typical (only) of the people who experienced the phenomenon at that particular time and place?[16] Further, if we permit ourselves to infer that the common meanings are genuinely intrinsic to the phenomenon, are we not ... well, generalising? Aren't we saying that *everyone else* who experiences the phenomenon – at whatever time, at whatever place – will attach the same meanings to it (because those meanings *belong to* the phenomenon)? And isn't generalisation supposed to be something PQR writers abstain from?

Second, is it not likely that the common meanings will be 'lowest common denominator' meanings (so to speak)? Won't they tend towards the trite, the predictable, the uninformative? In trying to identify meanings in such a way that they are characteristic of everybody in the sample, won't we end up with categories that are very general? Consider, for example, the study of people on haemodialysis by Moran *et al.* (2010), in which the 'overarching pattern' (as noted above) was 'waiting for a kidney transplant'. Does this come as a major surprise? Most people have haemodialysis precisely *because* they are waiting for kidney transplants, so the fact that they all mentioned this 'waiting' aspect during the interview is not particularly revealing. Identifying it as the 'overarching pattern' certainly does not count as 'uncovering hidden meaning'. In attempting to find a 'pattern' that applies to everyone in the sample, Moran *et al.* have come up with a concept so wide that it is uninformative: it simply repeats what we already know about the reasons for being on haemodialysis in the first place. If this is intrinsic meaning, it's not very interesting.

As the discussion progresses, it becomes evident that 'meaning intrinsic to the phenomenon' is not in itself a very clear idea, although some methodologists (especially Giorgi and van Manen) seem to treat it as unproblematic. In later chapters, then, I will be interested in their reasons for thinking that meaning *is* an attribute of phenomena, and in their methods for determining what that meaning is in any particular case.

Description or interpretation?

When introducing the three types of conclusion in qualitative studies, I used a deliberately neutral term, 'conclusion', to refer to the summary statement arising out of data analysis. My purpose in adopting this term was to avoid prejudging the question as to whether this summary statement is purely a *description* or whether it is an *interpretation*. Obviously, phenomenologists squabble about this. Those of a broadly Husserlian persuasion (Giorgi) insist that PQR must restrict itself to describing, while those of a rather more Heideggerian bent (van Manen; Smith *et al.*) argue that interpreting is not merely permissible but inevitable.

This sometimes appears akin to the debate between Big-Endians and Little-Endians because, from one point of view, both description and interpretation are such unambitious activities. PQR researchers are forbidden from taking an interest in causes and consequences, models and mechanisms, but why is this? What reasons are offered for sticking to describing (or interpreting) when there are so many other more interesting things one might be doing? Do PQR writers ever wonder about this? Do they understand why phenomenology is an 'interpretive method' (or a 'descriptive method'), and why the alternatives are off limits? Do they accept that it is illegitimate to explain, theorise, model, test, hypothesise, evaluate, infer, simulate ... and, if so, on what grounds? What justifies this kind of flat reductionism – the idea that the world consists of nothing but 'phenomena' awaiting 'description' or 'interpretation'?

Both descriptivists and interpretivists are in the business of attaching predicates to the phenomenon: its meaning is this, its essence is that, its nature is the other, its lived structure is something else. This is, I have suggested, what distinguishes PQR from other qualitative genres; so it is futile to argue (here) that it should adopt an alternative goal: explaining, theorising, modelling, hypothesising, testing, evaluating, and so on. I will leave that until the last chapter. My point is, rather, that descriptivists and interpretivists are unambitious in the same way; and it is this shared lack of ambition that makes the disputes between them faintly ridiculous.

However, this debate does pose another question for the book's agenda. What exactly is the difference between 'description' and 'interpretation'? In PQR, how do we know whether a particular conclusion is descriptive or interpretive? Obviously, the researcher will have a view about this, and will no doubt say what it is. But are there any indicators? Is there something about how the conclusion is formulated that tells the reader 'this is a description' or 'this is an interpretation'? If the author didn't tell you, would you still know? If so, on what basis? How well defined is the distinction in the first place? For example, one PQR researcher's conclusion is that:

> Jealousy is experienced in a situation where P is not receiving sufficient attention and appreciation for herself and another person actively *robs* P of the *already lacking* attention and appreciation desired by P.
>
> (Giorgi 2009)

Is this a *description* of jealousy or an *interpretation* of it? Whatever your answer, do you know just by looking at it? If it is a description, what does it mean to say that a person has robbed someone else of something she doesn't have? Doesn't that look suspiciously like a rather paradoxical interpretation?[17] Or consider an earlier example: according to Moran *et al.* (2010), the 'overarching pattern' associated with haemodialysis is 'waiting for a kidney transplant'. This is presumably intended as an interpretation, because the study is an example of 'Heideggerian phenomenology', and the 'data were analysed using a qualitative interpretive approach'. But to describe somebody on haemodialysis as waiting for a kidney transplant ... isn't that just a straightforward description? Well, perhaps someone will argue that it isn't. But, if not, in what sense is it an interpretation? And how can we tell the difference?

It is not often that questions of this sort are acknowledged by PQR authors. It is even less often that an attempt is made to answer them.

The axiom of resident meaning

I have suggested that PQR is distinguished from other qualitative genres by its commitment to meaning attribution. Its primary aim is to attribute meaning to the phenomenon as a whole, and it achieves this by attributing meaning to individual units of data. However, there is one serious qualification (hybrids) and a number of not-usually-answered questions still in the pending tray.

Figure 2.3 presents a schema of the phenomenological picture. We begin with a phenomenon, which some people have experienced. By interviewing a sample of these people, the researcher generates data about the phenomenon. During data analysis, she attributes meaning to individual data units, and (by means of a procedure yet to be examined) arrives at a statement that attributes meaning to the phenomenon as a whole. Despite the qualifications and unanswered questions, this picture is a reasonably accurate sketch of what PQR authors have in mind. The primary problem is that we do not have much idea how the meaning attributions are carried out because the vast majority of accounts are so cursory.

This picture suggests one final question that I want to consider before closing the chapter: Where does the meaning come from? When the researcher proposes a meaning attribution, is she distilling something that already exists (as it were) in the data? Or is she making essential use of some external resource such as a theory? To change the metaphor: is the meaning *resident* in the text being analysed, or is it derived from something external to the text?

It should be noted that this question is different from the one discussed earlier: whether the meaning is intrinsic or attached. That was a question about whether meaning was a property of the *phenomenon*. The question about residence concerns what can be inferred (and on what basis) from the *data*. It is the difference, if you like, between an ontological question ('Is meaning a property of phenomena?') and an epistemological question ('Is meaning inferred from the data/text alone, or must some other source be invoked?'). In principle, there are four possible positions:

i   meaning is a property of the phenomenon, and it is inferred from the text alone;
ii   meaning is a property of the phenomenon, but is inferred from a source external to the data;
iii meaning is attached to the phenomenon by respondents, but it must be inferred from an external source;
iv   meaning is attached to the phenomenon, but must be inferred from the text alone.

Giorgi adopts position (i); Smith *et al.* adopt position (iv); van Manen for the most part adopts position (i), but sometimes seems to veer towards position (iv).[18]

Unlike the other questions outlined in this chapter, the 'resident meaning' question is answered clearly by the three texts I'll be examining. Despite differences in their interpretation of the phenomenological tradition, all three methodological authors have the same epistemological view. Indeed, it is stated explicitly as a fundamental principle of their work. I call this principle the *axiom of resident meaning*.

The axiom of resident meaning says: the meaning that is attributed to a text by an interpreter does not come from anywhere other than the text itself. It is (in some sense) *resident* in the text, although it is (in some sense) also *hidden* in the text, and

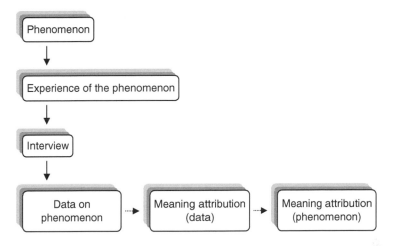

Figure 2.3 The phenomenological picture.

has to be formulated by an expert interpreter, who illuminates, elucidates, uncovers, unearths, understands, distils, or otherwise retrieves the meaning.

For example, SFL suggest: the interpretation 'is not usually based on importing a reading from without' (37). Rather, interpretation must be 'based on a reading from within the text itself', 'a close reading of what is already in the passage' (105). IPA does not take a theory from external sources – one example mentioned by the authors is psychoanalysis – and then make the data fit. Connections can be made to an external theory *afterwards*, but the 'internal', based-entirely-on-the-text analysis must come first.

Giorgi and van Manen take the same view. Giorgi says: 'a descriptive analysis attempts to understand the meaning of the description based solely on what is present in the data' (127). Van Manen says that: 'the meaning or essence of a phenomenon' is grasped by coming to grips 'with the structure of meaning of the text', examining every sentence and asking: 'What does this sentence ... reveal about the phenomenon or experience being described?' (78, 93). For all three writers, the meaning of the phenomenon (or experience) is somehow embedded in the data/text. External sources, and particularly external theory, are out.

Paradoxically, perhaps, the meaning is also hidden in the text. From one point of view, this is inevitable. If it were not hidden, one would not (presumably) need an expert to elucidate it. As van Manen (2014) notes: 'what "appears" is not at all something apparent or clear-given. If it were, then phenomenology would not be necessary: we would simply see what it is that "appears"' (61). However, if we ask *how* and *why* the meaning of 'what appears' is hidden – for what reason the phenomenon 'largely hides itself (its lived meanings) in its appearance' – the answer is not so straightforward.

Often, an appeal is made to Heidegger (1962) at this point, and to the idea that the phenomenon can be subject to a 'covering-up' in the sense of 'hiddenness, burying-over, or disguise' (36). It is not obvious that, without a great deal of exegesis, this explains very much. So, for the sake of argument, I propose to accept that the meaning of a phenomenon is both *resident* and *hidden* in the text. It is possible that, when we begin to study examples of PQR analysis more closely, it will become clear exactly what kind of hiddenness this is.

However, we still do not know (if we rely on published research reports) how this resident-but-hidden meaning can be uncovered. Methodologically speaking, this is the most important question. The other questions discussed in this chapter have philosophical significance, and some may have methodological ramifications. But the question as to how meaning attribution is achieved – how the analysis of the data/text is actually carried out – is critical. If we don't understand that, how can we claim to have undertaken a PQR study? How can we pretend to evaluate one? We can argue about what kind of meaning the PQR researcher is trying to distil, and what it is that she attributes meaning to – the phenomenon ready to shine forth, or the contents of consciousness. But these issues do not have a direct bearing on analytical practice. An understanding of how meaning attribution is actually accomplished ... does.

In the next two chapters, therefore, I will turn to the methodological texts by Giorgi and van Manen, and examine the extended examples of phenomenological analysis that they provide. The hope is that by studying these examples closely we will be able to determine how meaning attribution works.

Notes

1 Recent examples include: Gibson and Watkins (2012); Giske and Cone (2012); Van Dover and Pfeiffer (2012); Helgesen *et al.* (2013); Reisenhofer and Seibold (2013); Dlugasch and Ugarriza (2014); Førsund *et al.* (2015); Lee *et al.* (2014).
2 Norlyk and Harder (2010) ask the same question differently: What makes a phenomenological study phenomenological? To answer it, they review 37 papers (published during 2006–7) which had a nurse as first author. Their conclusion: 'The variations, apparent inconsistencies, and omissions make it unclear what makes a phenomenological study phenomenological' (429). They recommend that published studies based on phenomenology 'should include a minimum of scientific criteria', which is a good idea; and that 'it is important to clarify how the principles of phenomenological philosophy are implemented in a particular study', which probably isn't.
3 There is an ambiguity in 'common' that is rarely discussed. It can mean 'frequent', as in 'frosts are common this time of year'; or it can mean 'universal', as in 'some physiological mechanisms are common to all mammals'. So are 'common themes' common in the frequency sense? Do they turn up in *many* (but not all) of the transcripts? Or are they common in the universal sense? Do they turn up in *all* the transcripts? Which of these different senses is intended by qualitative researchers is not always clear. However, the ambiguity does not affect the point I am making in the text.
4 There are the makings here of an argument against the polarisation of qualitative and quantitative research. Crudely, qualitative research implies categorisation, or at any rate most forms of it do. But if you can categorise, you can count. Create categories, assign units of data to them, then count the number of units in each category. Some categories will have higher observed frequencies than others. You might not *want* to count, for various ideological reasons. But if you have created categories, then you have put yourself – willy-nilly, like it or not – in a position where counting is possible.

To that extent, counting and categorisation are just opposite sides of the same coin. And this is only one of the reasons why the distinction between qualitative and quantitative should not be exaggerated. Further discussion, from different angles, can be found in Paley (2000, 2010).

5 There is no need for 'causal' to frighten the horses here. It is intended only in the sense of one thing leading to another, one thing bringing about another, or one thing prompting another. There are no scary deterministic implications. 'The fact that it was very cold prompted me to put a fleece on before going outside' is a causal statement. The world, including the human world, is dense with things leading to other things, and there is no way we can abstain from using such concepts, even though they are causal. Resistance to the idea of causation in the human world is based on an extremely narrow view of what causation is. Illari and Russo (2014) is an excellent primer.

6 Of course, we do not know what the gradient of the graph would be, because we do not know what the precise value of *f* is. We don't even know if the the line mapping the relation is straight or curved (if *f* defines a nonlinear relation, it will be curved). But whatever the details, it will be true that *more x* is associated with *more y*. This is the basic claim Glaser and Strauss made: the greater the social loss (*x*), the better the care (*y*). You don't have to specify the exact values in suggesting that the relation between *x* and *y* is of this kind.

7 It would take too long to explain the difference between these terms; and for the purposes of this chapter it is not crucial. However, it does not require much reflection to see that, usually, the 'meaning' of X and the 'essence' of X are not identical. The *essence* of water, for example, is presumably H_2O. The *meaning* of water might refer to the pleasures of sailing or swimming, its significance in certain religions (baptism), and so on. For an account of the debate about essences in philosophy of science, see Slater and Borghini (2011).

8 It would be helpful to know how 'contributory' and 'disruptive' are operationalised. Exactly what does a 'contributory' interaction look like, and what indicators are used to measure it? Unfortunately, the Glenn *et al.* paper is uninformative in this respect. But their thesis can still be construed as a hypothesis about the link between certain interventions and patient outcomes. However, before the hypothesis could confidently be taken as a basis for action, the variables would have to be operationalised, and the model would need to be tested.

9 Nor is this the end of it. The *Discussion* (2880–2882) emphasises the consultants' understanding of CNC/CMC practice as 'wide-ranging and all inclusive', contrasted to 'conventional expectations, driven largely by uncompromising bureaucratic management approaches'. It points to the participants' 'leadership and intellectual skills', the way they provide 'clear direction', motivate others and facilitate change. They also have a 'propensity to anticipate the unexpected and discern and forestall potential impediments to effective care delivery'. In addition, they are capable of seeing 'the bigger picture' and 'transcending traditional expectations and obstacles'. They tend to 'use a non-confrontational approach', and have 'developed a flexible leadership style'. However, they 'encounter barriers from others who are unaware' of this. They have an 'explicit understanding of gaps in service provision', and their passion is 'nurtured by their implicit motivation', and by their 'authentic caring'. They have 'personal resilience' and 'personal bravery' when their clinical effectiveness is threatened; and they are willing to 'speak up when under pressure'. They are 'facilitators of the patient's own authentic consciousness'. They act as 'self-motivated visionary change agents who are prepared to take risks'.

10 Of course, the reference to 'reflection' is an attempt to persuade the reader that the author is aware of the possibility of spurious conjecture, and has taken steps to reduce the risk that she will succumb. 'Our assumptions and pre-understandings were explicated by our openness and reflection' is condensed code for: 'by reflecting on our own thinking, and by being open to the possibility that we were projecting our own ideas

into the data, we identified the assumptions and presuppositions that we brought to the topic, and which might have turned out to be wrong'. It is not clear, from this brief description, what the point of the 'openness and reflection' manoeuvre is in this particular case.

Some authors (usually those who talk of 'bracketing') say that, having identified their presuppositions, they can disable them, as if toggling them to 'off'. I have a problem with this: I do not understand how either of the two steps can be achieved. In the first place, how do I identify the relevant presuppositions? Is it not likely that the ones which exert most influence on my thinking will be unconscious, or at least very difficult to retrieve? Is it possible to identify these presuppositions by introspection? If so, how? How does it work? What do I have to do? If not, what other psychological process is involved? In the second place, how can the presuppositions, once identified, be turned off? Is this a kind of ignoring? If so, how convincing can it be to assure the reader that my preconceptions and prejudices have played no part in the analysis because I have ignored them? What evidence of that can I provide? If it is not a kind of ignoring, what else is it?

A second group of authors imply that, if they set out their preconceptions, the reader will be able to 'allow' for them, so to speak, when studying the paper, as if the reader can 'subtract' the presuppositions from the researcher's text, and 'weight' the findings accordingly. I have yet to see an account of how the reader is supposed to do this. A third group refuses to play the 'identifying presuppositions' game, and accepts that any analysis will be a function of the author's preconceptions. That's just how it is, take it or leave it. Given their own premises, this is an admirably logical strategy. My problem, in this case, is that I do not see how what they say about the study can serve as a basis for doing anything (clinically, or in policy terms) on the basis of the findings. If what the researcher tells me is basically a reflection of her own prejudices, why does that give *me* a reason for action?

11 The ambiguity in this case is different from van Manen's ambiguity, discussed earlier. Van Manen is ambiguous about what *property* of the phenomenon he seeks to identify (meaning, essence, nature, or whatever). SFL are ambiguous about *what kind of thing* this property is a property *of* (the thing itself, lived experience, the phenomenon ready to shine forth, and so on).

12 Useful discussions of how phenomena are identified in science can be found in Bailer-Jones (2009) and Craver and Darden (2013). Both argue that prior causal knowledge is necessary in order to define a phenomenon in the first place, and that phenomena are often *redefined* as a result of empirical enquiry (because a revised understanding of causal processes implies new ways of demarcating one phenomenon from another). I return to this topic in Chapter 7.

13 The best discussion of 'experience' that I know of is Wierzbicka (2010), who discusses the history of the word using corpus linguistics. She shows that the focus on 'experience' is Anglocentric: no other European language has a word that is its direct equivalent. According to Wierzbicka, 'experience' has seven senses, including: (a) situation/event that someone observes or undergoes; (b) an awareness-cum-feeling that someone has at a particular time. I suggest a comparable distinction in Paley (2014b).

PQR researchers who claim to explore the experience of such-and-such a group rarely distinguish between these two senses. Consequently, there is a characteristic PQR 'slide'. During the philosophical and methodological discussion, researchers emphasise that phenomenology is concerned with subjective experience, and takes no interest in objective events and circumstances. However, by the time they get to the 'recommendations' section, they appear to have forgotten this, because their proposals are based on the assumption that the respondents' accounts are a reliable guide to things that actually happened.

This is a slide from 'studying the subjective-experience-of-X' to 'drawing conclusions about X'. I give examples in Paley (2005). Here are three more recent ones.

Hughes *et al.* (2010) slide from claiming that their respondents do not *recall* being informed about the aftermath of surgery to assuming that *in reality* their information needs were unmet. Scheckel *et al.* (2010) slide from eight nursing students' self-reports on the experience of providing patient education, to assertions about 'the extraordinary competencies students already have in addressing health literacy'. Ranheim *et al.* (2010) slide from nurses' subjective experiences of providing patients with rhythmical embrocation to claims that 'the participating nurses' sensitivity and abilities in observation grew wider and more receptive'. In all cases, the researchers drift from their official position, according to which they restrict themselves to their respondents' subjective perceptions, to the assumption that these perceptions correspond to what objectively occurred.

14 Murphy (2010) is an excellent introduction to lexical meaning.

15 To which van Manen (2014) adds embedded meaning, experiential meaning, felt meaning, iconic meaning, poetic meaning, existential meaning, lifeworld meaning, special meaning, original meaning, non-cognitive meaning, and evoked meaning ... among others.

16 'Saturation' is the most popular answer to this question. The idea is that, if you are not eliciting any new types of response by, say, the eighth interview, you can strike camp and go home because you have unearthed all the relevant categories associated with this phenomenon. However, saturation only makes sense in the context of theoretical sampling (Glaser and Strauss 1967), or some other strategy designed to test the current analysis to destruction by increasing the probability that it will fail. Which is why Glaser and Strauss constantly emphasise the selection of maximally different settings. As they say, the researcher 'goes out of his way to look for groups that stretch diversity of data as far as possible'. 'Saturation', in other words, means no-new-categories-despite-several-energetic-attempts-to-show-that-the-current-set-of-categories-is-inadequate. By contrast, concluding a series of interviews because a handful of self-selecting respondents from the same setting have generated all the categories there are to be found is just wishful thinking. This watering down of 'saturation' is another consequence of QRAS, since production-line postgraduate students usually do not have the time or the resources to pursue theoretical sampling.

17 This is the first part of Barbro Giorgi's version of the 'structure of jealousy', to be found in Giorgi (2009). Presumably, then, it is intended to be a description, since Giorgi's phenomenological method is explicitly descriptive. My question is this: if you didn't already know that this account of 'jealousy' is supposed to be a descriptive one, would you be able to tell?

18 My own view, which will become clear later in the book, does not fit this typology. But it is closer to position (iii) than to any of the others.

References

Atsalos, C., Biggs, K., Boensch, S., Gavegan, F. L., Heath, S., Payk, M., and Trapolini, G. (2014) 'How clinical nurse and midwifery consultants optimise patient care in a tertiary referral hospital', *Journal of Clinical Nursing*, 23, pp. 2874–2885.

Bailer-Jones, D. (2009) *Scientific Models in Philosophy of Science*. Pittsburgh, PA: University of Pittsburgh Press.

Burhans, L. M., and Alligood, M. R. (2010) 'Quality nursing care in the words of nurses', *Journal of Advanced Nursing*, 66(8), pp. 1689–1697.

Charmaz, K. (2014) *Constructing Grounded Theory*. 2nd Edition. London: Sage.

Cheng, C.-H., Wang, T.-J., Lin, Y.-P., Lin, H.-R., Hu, W.-Y., Wung, S.-H., and Liang, S.-Y. (2013) 'The illness experience of middle-aged men with oral cancer', *Journal of Clinical Nursing*, 22, pp. 3549–3556.

Cohen, M. Z. (1987) 'A historical overview of the phenomenological movement', *Image: Journal of Nursing Scholarship*, 19(1), pp. 31–34.

Craver, C. F., and Darden, L. (2013) *In Search of Mechanisms: Discoveries Across the Life Sciences.* Chicago: University of Chicago Press.

Creswell, J. D. (2003) *Research Design: Qualitative, Quantitative and Mixed Method Approaches.* 2nd edition. Thousand Oaks: Sage.

Crotser, C. B., and Dickerson, S. S. (2010) 'Women receiving news of a family BRCA 1/2 mutation: messages of fear and empowerment', *Journal of Nursing Scholarship*, 42(4), pp. 367–378.

Dlugasch, L. B., and Ugarriza, D. N. (2014) 'Self-monitoring of blood glucose experiences of adults with type 2 diabetes', *Journal of the American Association of Nurse Practitioners*, 26(6), pp. 323–329.

Elmir, R., Jackson, D., Beale, B., and Schmied, V. (2010) 'Against all odds: Australian women's experiences of recovery from breast cancer', *Journal of Clinical Nursing*, 19, pp. 2531–2538.

Ernersson, Å., Lindtsröm, T., Nyström, F. H., and Frisman, G. H. (2010) 'Young healthy individuals develop lack of energy when adopting an obesity-provoking behaviour for 4 weeks: a phenomenological analysis', *Scandinavian Journal of Caring Sciences*, 24, pp. 565–571.

Førsund, L. H., Skovdahl, K., Kiik, R., and Ytrehus, S. (2015) 'The loss of a shared lifetime: a qualitative study exploring spouses' experiences of losing couplehood with their partner with dementia living in institutional care', *Journal of Clinical Nursing*, 24(1–2), pp. 121–130.

Furseth, I. (2005) 'From "Everything has a meaning" to "I want to believe in something": religious change between two generations of women in Norway', *Social Compass*, 52(2), pp. 157–168.

Galvin, G., and Timmins, F. (2010) 'A phenomenological exploration of intellectual disability: nurse's experiences of managerial support', *Journal of Nursing Management*, 18(6), pp. 726–735.

Gibson, J., and Watkins, C. (2012) 'People's experiences of the impact of transient ischaemic attack and its consequences: qualitative study', *Journal of Advanced Nursing*, 68(8), pp. 1707–1715.

Giorgi, A. (1985) 'Sketch of a psychological phenomenological method', in A. Giorgi (ed.) *Phenomenology and Psychological research.* Pittsburgh: Duquesne University Press, pp. 8–22.

Giorgi, A. (1997) 'The theory, practice and evaluation of the phenomenological method as a qualitative research procedure', *Journal of Phenomenological Psychology*, 28(2), pp. 235–260.

Giorgi, A. (2009) *The Descriptive Phenomenological Method in Psychology: A Modified Husserlian Approach.* Pittsburgh: Duquesne University Press.

Giske, T., and Cone, P. H. (2012) 'Opening up to learning spiritual care of patients: a grounded theory study of nursing students', *Journal of Clinical Nursing*, 21(13–14), pp. 2006–2015.

Glaser, B. G., and Strauss, A. L. (1967) *The Discovery of Grounded Theory: Strategies for Qualitative research.* New Brunswick: Aldine Transaction.

Glenn, L. A., Stocker-Schnieder, J., McCune, R., McClelland, M., and King, D. (2014) 'Caring nurse practice in the intrapartum setting: nurses' perspectives on complexity, relationships and safety', *Journal of Advanced Nursing*, 70(9), pp. 2019–2030.

Greenfield, G., Pliskin, J. S., Feder-Bubis, P., Wientroub, S., and Davidovitch, N. (2012) 'Patient-physician relationships in second opinion encounters: the physicians' perspective', *Social Science and Medicine*, 75(7), pp. 1202–1212.

Hammersley, M. (1992) *What's Wrong With Ethnography?* London: Routledge.

Hansson, K. S., Fridlund, B., Brunt, D., Hansson, B., and Rask, M. (2011) 'The meaning of the experiences of persons with chronic pain in their encounters with the health service', *Scandinavian Journal of Caring Studies*, 25(3), pp. 444–450.

Heidegger, M. (1962) *Being and Time*. Oxford: Basil Blackwell.

Helgesen, A. K., Larsson, M., and Athlin, E. (2013) 'How do relatives of persons with dementia experience their role in the patient participation process in special care units', *Journal of Clinical Nursing*, 22(11–12), pp. 1672–1681.

Herlin, C., and Wann-Hansson, C. (2010) 'The experience of being 30–45 years of age and depending on haemodialysis treatment: a phenomenological study', *Scandinavian Journal of Caring Sciences*, 24(4), pp. 693–699.

Holloway, I., and Wheeler, S. (2010) *Qualitative Research in Nursing and Healthcare*. 3rd edition. Oxford: Wiley-Blackwell.

Hughes, C., Knibb, W., and Allan, H. (2010) 'Laparoscopic surgery for endometrial cancer: a phenomenological study', *Journal of Advanced Nursing*, 66(11), pp. 2500–2509.

Illari, P., and Russo, F. (2014) *Causality: Philosophical Theory Meets Scientific Practice*. Oxford: Oxford University Press.

Kornhaber, R., Wilson, A., Abu-Qamar, M., McLean, L., and Vandervord, J. (2015) 'Inpatient peer support for adult burn survivors: a valuable resource: a phenomenological analysis of the Australian experience', *Burns*, 41(1), pp. 110–117.

Kouwenhoven, S. E., Kirkevold, M., Engedal, K., and Kim, H. S. (2011) '"Living a life in shades of grey": experiencing depressive symptoms in the acute phase after stroke', *Journal of Advanced Nursing*, 68(8), pp. 1726–1737.

Lee, P.-S., Lee, C.-L., Hu, S.-T., and Tasao, L.-I. (2014) 'Relieving my discomforts safely: the experiences of discontinuing HRT among menopausal women', *Journal of Clinical Nursing*, 23(17–18), pp. 2481–2490.

Lindy, C., and Schaefer, F. (2010) 'Negative workplace behaviours: an ethical dilemma for nurse managers', *Journal of Nursing Management*, 18(3), pp. 285–292.

Little, C. V. (2012) 'Patient expectations of "effectiveness" in health care: an example from medical herbalism', *Journal of Clinical Nursing*, 21(5–6), pp. 718–727.

Maxwell, J. A. (2012) *A Realist Approach for Qualitative Research*. Thousand Oaks, CA: Sage.

Monaro, S., Stewart, G., and Gullick, J. (2014) 'A "lost life": coming to terms with haemodialysis', *Journal of Clinical Nursing*, 23(21–22), pp. 3262–3273.

Moran, A., Scott, A., and Darbyshire, P. (2010) 'Waiting for a kidney transplant: patients' experiences of haemodialysis therapy', *Journal of Advanced Nursing*, 67(3), pp. 501–509.

Morse, J. M., and Field, P. A. (1995) *Qualitative Research Methods for Health Professionals*. 2nd edition. Thousand Oaks, CA: Sage.

Murphy, M. L. (2010) *Lexical Meaning*. Cambridge, UK: Cambridge University Press.

Norlyk, A., and Harder, I. (2010) 'What makes a phenomenological study phenomenological? An analysis of peer-reviewed empirical nursing studies', *Qualitative Health Research*, 20(3), pp. 420–431.

Ødbehr, L. S., Kvigne, K., Hauge, S., and Danbolt, L. J. (2015) 'A qualitative study of nurses' attitudes towards and accommodations of patients' expressions of religiosity and faith in dementia care', *Journal of Advanced Nursing*, 71(2), pp. 359–369.

Paley, J. (2000) 'Paradigms and presuppositions: the difference between qualitative and quantitative research', *Scholarly Inquiry for Nursing Practice*, 14(2), pp. 143–155.

Paley, J. (2005) 'Phenomenology as rhetoric', *Nursing Inquiry*, 12(2), pp. 106–116.

Paley, J. (2010) 'Qualitative interviewing as measurement', *Nursing Philosophy*, 11(2), 112–126.

Paley, J. (2014) 'Heidegger, lived experience and method', *Journal of Advanced Nursing*, 70(7), pp. 1520–1531.

Paley, J. (2016) 'Evidence and the qualitative research analogous structure', in M. Lipscomb (ed.) *Exploring Evidence-based Practice: Debates and Challenges in Nursing*. Abingdon, UK: Routledge, pp. 132–150.

Parahoo, K. (2014) *Nursing Research: Principles, Process and Issues*. 3rd edition. Basingstoke, UK: Palgrave Macmillan.

Pawson, R., and Tilley, N. (1997) *Realistic Evaluation*. London: Sage.

Phillips, J., and Cohen, M. Z. (2011) 'The meaning of breast cancer risk for African American women', *Journal of Nursing Scholarship*, 43(3), pp. 239–247.

Ranheim, A., Kärner, A., Arman, M., Rehnsfeldt, A. W., and Berterö, C. (2010) 'Embodied reflection in practice – "touching the core of caring"', *International Journal of Nursing Practice*, 16(3), pp. 241–247.

Reisenhofer, S., and Seibold, C. (2013) 'Emergency healthcare experiences of women living with intimate partner violence', *Journal of Clinical Nursing*, 22(15–16), pp. 2253–2263.

Repstad, P. (2009) 'A softer God and a more positive anthropology: changes in a religiously strict region in Norway', *Religion*, 39(2), pp. 126–131.

Scheckel, M., Emery, N., and Nosek, C. (2010) 'Addressing health literacy: the experiences of undergraduate nursing students', *Journal of Clinical Nursing*, 19(5–6), pp. 794–802.

Silverman, D. (2000) *Doing Qualitative Research: A Practical Handbook*. London: Sage.

Slater, M. H., and Borghini, A. (2011) 'Introduction: lessons from the scientific butchery', in J. K. Campbell, M. O'Rourke, and M. H. Slater (eds.) *Carving Nature At Its Joints: Natural Kinds in Metaphysics and Science*. Cambridge, MA: MIT Press, pp. 1–31.

Smith, J. A., Flowers, P., and Larkin, M. (2009) *Interpretative Phenomenological Analysis*. London: Sage.

Sparrow, T. (2014) *The End of Phenomenology: Metaphysics and the New Realism*. Edinburgh: Edinburgh University Press.

Tavakol, S., Dennick, R., and Tavakol, M. (2012) 'Medical students' understanding of empathy: a phenomenological study', *Medical Education*, 46(3), pp. 306–316.

Thorkildsen, K., and Råholm, M.-B. (2010) 'The essence of professional competence experienced by Norwegian nurse students: a phenomenological study', *Nurse Education in Practice*, 10(4), pp. 183–188.

Thurang, A., Fagerberg, I., Palmstierna, T., and Tops, A. B. (2010) 'Women's experiences of caring when in treatment for alcohol dependency', *Scandinavian Journal of Caring Sciences*, 24(4), pp. 700–706.

Torresan, M. M., Garrino, L., Borraccino, A., Macchi, G., De Luca, A., and Dimonte, V. (2015) 'Adherence to treatment in patient with severe cancer pain: a qualitative enquiry through illness narratives', *European Journal of Oncology Nursing*, 19(4), pp. 397–404.

Van Dover, L., and Pfeiffer, J. (2012) 'Patients of parish nurses experience renewed spiritual identity: a grounded theory study', *Journal of Advanced Nursing*, 68(8), pp. 1824–1844.

van Manen, M. (1990) *Researching Lived Experience: Human Science for an Action Sensitive Pedagogy.* Albany, NY: State University of New York Press.

van Manen, M. (2014) *Phenomenology of Practice: Meaning-Giving Methods in Phenomenological Research and Writing.* Walnut Creek, CA: Left Coast Press.

Vuori, A., and Åstedt-Kurki, P. (2013) 'Experiences of health and well-being among Finnish low-income fathers', *Nursing Inquiry*, 20(2), pp. 165–175.

Waller, J., and Pattison, N. (2013) 'Men's experiences of regaining urinary contintence following robotic-assisted laparoscopic prostatectomy (RALP) for localised prostate cancer: a qualitative phenomenological study', *Journal of Clinical Nursing*, 22(3–4), pp. 368–378.

Wierzbicka, A. (2010) *Experience, Evidence, and Sense: The Hidden Cultural Legacy of English.* Oxford: Oxford University Press.

Wilson, A. M. E. (2014) 'Application of Heideggerian phenomenology to mentorship of nursing students', *Journal of Advanced Nursing*, 70(12), pp. 2910–2919.

Zuckerman, P. (2007) 'Atheism: contemporary numbers and patterns', in M. Martin (ed.) *The Cambridge Companion to Atheism.* Cambridge, UK: Cambridge University Press, pp. 47–65.

3 Amedeo Giorgi
Jealousy

The last chapter of Amedeo Giorgi's (2009) book provides a detailed example of PQR (which he calls 'scientific phenomenology') in action.[1] The method described during the preceding pages of the book is used to arrive at an essential structure of jealousy, drawing on descriptions obtained from two workshop participants. The descriptions were written down by the participants concerned, and were then subject to analysis by two researchers, independently of each other. This is particularly interesting, as it permits Giorgi to compare the findings of two separate PQR researchers using the same method with the same data. The researchers in question are Giorgi himself (AG) and his late wife, Barbro Giorgi (BG).

Giorgi's chapter first sets out the two descriptions of jealousy in full, and then discusses the three main stages of the method (as conducted by AG and BG) in considerable detail. The account includes: (a) the identification of meaning units, in which the descriptions are segmented into a series of smaller chunks; (b) transformation, in which the meaning units are converted into more explicit expressions of meaning in 'language revelatory of the psychological aspect of the lived-through experience' (145); and lastly (c) the formulation of an essential structure of the phenomenon being researched, in this case jealousy. As the application of the method is traced in an equally detailed manner for each researcher, we have the opportunity to examine four sets of meaning units (two descriptions, each analysed by two researchers), four transformations (*ditto*), and two versions of the essential structure.

In this chapter, I propose to make use of this opportunity, and subject Giorgi's analysis (and that of BG) to close scrutiny. The primary focus, as explained in the last chapter, will be on meaning attribution.

The experience of jealousy

The two stories are reproduced below. The original descriptions are in Giorgi (2009: 140–142).

P_1

Some years ago, I was with a group of people in a three-day training. I had a casual friendship with some of them, and one of them I had just formed a very close friendship with. We are each happily married to our spouses, then and today. I do not feel attracted to my friend in a romantic way, but care deeply for him, as if he were my brother, as he does for me, then and today.

On the first full day of training, there was a lunch break. I had a cold and felt tired that morning. I knew I would not feel like walking to a nearby restaurant, so brought a snack. When it came time to break for lunch, my close friend turned to me to see what I was going to do. I told this person that the others were arranging a lunch together, but that I was going to stay in because I wasn't feeling well so brought some food. He decided to go out with the others, rather than stay in with me.

I understood why he decided to go with the others, because he didn't bring his lunch, but I really was secretly hoping he would stay in with me. It was perfectly reasonable that he would choose to go out but I felt hurt, and at the same time silly at having that feeling. When he left with them I was amazed at myself because I actually felt abandoned. It stung, as if I were in a snowstorm with the driving wind turning my cheeks red. It was both an emotional and a physical stinging. My heart ached with sorrow and disappointment that was far beyond what seemed like I should be feeling; after all, it was a new friendship. I really wanted to be with him.

Later it got worse. He didn't know any of the people in the lunch group that he went out with. I found out from other friends that were together with them, that one woman in the group was flirting with him over lunch. When they came back the same woman told me [that] she had an intense attraction to this man, and told him so at lunch. When we were all back in the group together, she continued to flirt with him. He looked at her in amazement, as did everyone.

I had images flash in my mind of pushing her out of the room and telling her to 'stop it'. It was a very strange feeling, something I don't experience often, and more aggressive than I ever remember feeling. I hoped that no one could see this was going on in me, but when I looked at her, then looked at him; looking at her as she flirted with him, I felt almost like standing up in a raging loss of self-control. It felt like I had energy pulsations coming up from my stomach into my chest, bursting with fire. Luckily, I managed to keep my composure and finished the day, amazed at myself for having such a negative and intense reaction to this woman.

P₂

Pam is perfect and I hate feeling this way. She doesn't really even know I exist except for the fact she can probably identify my picture if pressed to do so. Yet her every movement, thought and pursuit is the standard by which I judge all my own.

We are both in the fifth grade in a little country school with six grades and only 62 students. We are not friends or enemies. She's part Cherokee, and it is the Native American blood in her that colours her straight, shiny hair black, skin light brown, and eyes as black as her hair. She looks different than all of us in our largely German-Scandinavian community. I admire her difference, but it really bugs me that everyone else does too, to the degree that no one else seems to be special when she is around.

She doesn't even need to try to get attention. All she has to do is stand there and her appearance does it for her. I know it doesn't have anything to do with the fact that she is a good student, especially pretty, remarkably kind, and naturally thoughtful. Even if she were a witch everyone would prefer her over others anyway, because they do even before she opens her mouth.

The worst moment in this secret jealousy is right now – at school pet day. Among the assortment of yapping dogs, cats, tadpoles and hamsters, Pam's gleaming brown quarter horse literally and figuratively stand[s] head and shoulders above the rest. Being a country school, there are fields on all sides of us as well as a large pasture attached to the school for field days.

Pam stands in one of these fields in front of her horse holding its reins while it is being saddled. I am stunned. The entire school, with the exception of me, runs to stand near her, gazing at her without making any sound. 'It just figures', I whisper to myself. As if she didn't already have it all, she has to show up with a horse. My parent had said no to one, even though we own barns, pastures, and our own grain supply. I take my little dog to a bench and stay away from the 'fan club' that surrounds her. How could life be so unfair?

I try not to look, but I am just like the rest. I can't help but watch. The scene is beautiful, with a turquoise blue sky curving overhead, wild flowers quivering in a cool breeze, and two beautiful spirits – each equally shiny black hair – standing quietly and patiently before us all.

As soon as the horse is ready to ride, Pam slips into the saddle with a practiced lightness. She turns the horse with gentleness and skill and canters it in a wide circle around the field. Her hair and the horse's mane flutter in the rushing air. The throng of schoolmates that stood to watch her earlier now runs behind her waving wildflowers. I can't stand it. Why can't that be me? It is all I can do not to cry.

Which phenomenon?

Giorgi says little about these descriptions, except that they 'were obtained in a workshop', and that they were 'written to begin with'. Both stories refer to events that occurred several years before (P_2's story is clearly a present-tense account of something that happened to her when she was a child). Immediately, this makes them vulnerable to the fallibilities of memory. It is not so much the fact that the events may be misremembered – though, at such a distance, this is not unlikely – as the possibility that the emotions associated with those events have been reinterpreted, reconfigured, re-narrativised. So it is necessary to bear in mind that Giorgi's analysis of 'jealousy' may be based on semi-fictional accounts of feelings that were experienced a long time ago. It is stretching it a bit to call this 'lived' experience.

It is odd that Giorgi never refers to the difficulty of analysing a 'phenomenon' based on descriptions of *long past* events. In an earlier chapter, he admits that there is always a possibility of 'slippage' between the experience and the reporting of it, but he appears not to recognise the seriousness of the problem, and dismisses it quickly. However, if memory is as unreliable as the evidence implies (Loftus 1979; Kassin *et al.* 2001; Schacter and Addis 2007; Holland and Kensinger 2010), searching for meaning in descriptions like this is a precarious business. Important aspects of the event itself and the emotions retrospectively attached to it may have been left out, and some parts of what has been included may be reconstructed or even imaginary. Even though the example is presented as a simple exercise, one would expect Giorgi to mention the risks of placing too much faith in an 'essential structure' derived from such unreliable data. But he doesn't.

The first question prompted by the stories is how the phenomenon is identified in the first place. How is the boundary drawn around 'jealousy'? What must be included, what must be omitted? What degree of specificity is required? How does Giorgi know that these accounts describe instances of jealousy and not some other 'phenomenon'? Does he allow for the possibility that they represent a mixture of jealousy and some other emotion? Might the stories refer to very specific types of jealousy rather than to jealousy in general? Does this matter? If so, does the 'phenomenon' need to be identified more narrowly, so that Giorgi's analysis would be an analysis of 'X' kind of jealousy and not of jealousy per se? Giorgi raises none of these questions, and one is left with the impression that he invited his participants to produce accounts of their experiences of jealousy, and then took what he was offered on trust. If that is true, then he effectively delegated the resolution of all these problems – identifying the 'phenomenon' of jealousy in the first place – to his subjects.

Let me explore three of these questions a little further. First, the question of whether the two stories are examples of generic jealousy, so to speak, or whether they illustrate a more specific form. Consider P_1's narrative. Everyone I have shown it to has commented, quite spontaneously, on what strikes them as an inconsistency between the claims made in the first paragraph – 'I do not feel attracted to my friend in a romantic way' – and the extreme emotion portrayed in the last two paragraphs particularly. This sounds very much like sexual jealousy, despite the initial denial, and seems incommensurate with a recently established platonic friendship. In any case, it is rather odd to suggest that one has 'just formed a very close friendship'. Close friendships develop gradually over time, and their onset cannot usually be dated and timed in the way that the start of a sexual relationship can be.

So, at the very least, there are grounds for scepticism here. The point is that Giorgi shows no interest in the *type* of jealousy being portrayed. Suppose the story does represent an example of specifically sexual jealousy. Can Giorgi then use it as a basis for deriving the 'essential structure' of jealousy in general? Is it not possible that the essential structure of jealousy – as he portrays it – will include characteristics that are typical of sexual jealousy but not of other kinds? The worrying thing is that Giorgi does not even ask the question.

Second, the question of whether the stories are exclusively about jealousy, or whether they incorporate other emotions too. Look at P_1's story again. On my reading, the first three paragraphs have nothing at all to do with jealousy. There is no-one to be jealous of, and the person towards whom the jealousy is eventually directed has not yet entered the story. Up to this point, the story is about hurt feelings, pure and simple. The emotional reaction still seems exaggerated, given the circumstances described in the first paragraph; but the situation is clearly one in which P_1 is upset because of something her friend has done (or not done). A common enough predicament; but hurt feelings prompted by somebody's action or inaction does not entail that the person concerned is 'jealous'. She is 'hurt and upset'. No other label is warranted. The final two paragraphs do justify the description 'jealousy', of course, as the flirtatious woman enters the picture.

So the question arises: should the analysis of jealousy include both parts of the story, or just the final two paragraphs? Giorgi's analysis (as we shall see) applies 'jealousy' to the whole story. He makes no distinction between the hurt occasioned by the friend's absence and the jealousy triggered by the flirt. The fact that, without the flirting portion of the story, the first three paragraphs would not have merited the description 'jealousy' does not seem to occur to him. However, it is obvious that the question about how to draw the boundary around the 'phenomenon' is a difficult one. If someone includes 'irrelevant' material when asked to tell a story about jealousy, do we include that material in the analysis? And, if not, on what basis do we judge it irrelevant? Giorgi gives no sign that he recognises the significance of such questions.

Third, the problem of whether the accounts describe jealousy or some other phenomenon. In this case, if P_2's story is compared with P_1's, a major difference becomes evident. As a phenomenological writer, Tellenbach (1974: 462), has pointed out: 'Wherever jealousy arises, something is in danger of being lost which I regard as belonging to me.... Envy, on the other hand, is always directed toward something that is *primarily* someone *else's*'. On this basis, P_1's account can be classified as a story of jealousy. P_2's account, however, is surely one of envy. P_2 is envious of Pam, who receives all the attention from her schoolmates. P_1 is jealous of the flirting woman, who presents a threat to the relationship with her new close friend.

Envy is a two-term relation in which A envies B. Jealousy, on the other hand, is a three-term relation in which A is jealous of B because the latter poses a threat to her relationship with C. As Cobb-Stevens (2003) suggests, jealousy involves the potential loss of something, especially a beloved's affections. In contrast, to be envious is 'to desire what is possessed by another'. In envy, someone else 'has it all'. In jealousy, someone else threatens to take away what is already mine. Giorgi briefly acknowledges this difference towards the end of the chapter, but dismisses it for reasons I will examine later. During the analysis, however, he is happy to accept the two accounts as examples of jealousy, without giving any thought to the possibility that some other emotion might be involved.

All three of these questions concern the initial specification of the 'phenomenon', and the problem of how to draw a conceptual boundary round it. How wide, or how narrow, should this boundary be? In Giorgi's presentation of his method, this question is not answered. He requested accounts of 'jealousy', but did not attempt to specify the concept he intended; nor did he enquire whether the stories he received were examples of it or not. As a result, he is presented with two different kinds of narrative. P_1's story is arguably about a particular type of jealousy; so the boundary is, in this respect, drawn too narrowly. Her story also incorporates other emotions, specifically hurt feelings. In that respect, the boundary is drawn too widely. P_2's story, meanwhile, concerns not jealousy but envy. The boundary round the phenomenon is doubly blurred by a confusion of the two.

Even before he starts, then, we have reason to wonder whether Giorgi's analysis will be an analysis, not of 'generic' jealousy, but of sexual-jealousy-combined-with-hurt-feelings-and-confused-with-envy. If it is, the analysis will be a bit of a mess.

This is the nightmare option, though, as far as Giorgi is concerned. There is no way of knowing whether P_1's story really is an account of sexual jealousy misrepresented as jealousy-in-general. But it is at least a distinct possibility; and the charge against Giorgi is not that he has got it wrong, but that he has not bothered to wonder. It seems not to have occurred to him that the boundary around the 'phenomenon' might have been drawn too narrowly. Consequently, he can have no idea what his phenomenological analysis is an analysis of.

The question as to how a phenomenon is identified, and how boundaries should be drawn between one phenomenon and another, will crop up throughout the book. It is of particular importance in Chapter 7.

Meaning units

The first step in Giorgi's method is to read the descriptions in order to get the overall sense. I am not going to say anything about this, except to observe that Giorgi says nothing about how 'overall sense' is determined. Why this might be a problem will become evident later.

The second is to break them into parts 'by establishing what are called "meaning units"' (142). He describes the procedure for achieving this as follows: 'Every time the researcher … experiences a shift of meaning in the description as he or she rereads it, a mark is made at that place in the description' (143). The researcher must adopt an attitude that synthesises 'the phenomenological reduction, a psychological perspective, and mindfulness of the fact that the description purports to be an experience of jealousy'. This sounds like skilled and subtle work, requiring an understanding of meaning, shifts of meaning, and the psychological perspective.

The fact that the 'meaning units' identified by both AG and BG are reproduced in the text gives us an opportunity to compare their attempts to carry out this procedure. The results are a little disappointing. As Giorgi concedes (179), 'we can see that they are not all identical. There are some commonalities and some differences'.

This is something of an understatement. A comparison of BG's units and AG's gives us Table 3.1:

Table 3.1 Meaning units in the two jealousy stories

BG's meaning units	P_1	P_2	Total
Correspond with AG's	9	10	19
Don't correspond with AGs	4	6	10

In other words, over a third of BG's meaning-unit 'marks' do not correspond to marks made by AG. Of the 19 that do correspond, eight coincide with paragraph endings, which seems a rather obvious place to put them. So, if we exclude those for a moment (as being too easy), nearly half of BG's unit markers fail to correspond to AG's.

In any case, this looks to be an unduly high proportion, given that both these analysts are 'experienced phenomenological researchers', applying a method that they presumably had plenty of opportunity to discuss. It would appear that identifying 'shifts in meaning' is not a particularly reliable process.

Giorgi himself is remarkably cavalier about this outcome. Having noted that there are major differences between AG's and BG's 'shift in meaning' markers, he suggests: 'This is to be expected ... whether they are the same or different does not matter' (179). This comes as a surprise in view of his claim that identifying 'shifts in meaning' requires an attitude that incorporates the 'phenomenological reduction, the psychological perspective, and mindfulness of the fact that the story purports to be an experience of jealousy' (ibid.). But his explanation of why the 'meaning unit/marker' differences between AG and BG don't matter is even more surprising. He now argues that 'this second step is a practical one and carries no theoretical weight' (ibid.). This is because 'the constitution of meaning units simply makes the analysis more feasible because it is difficult to retain the whole description in mind while doing detailed analyses' (ibid.). In other words, the sole purpose of breaking the stories into units is to reduce them to shorter, manageable segments. It is difficult remember the whole story during the analysis, so we have to break it into small chunks and take it one piece at a time. It's not a theoretical issue, it's just convenient.

So Giorgi has two mutually contradictory explanations of the process of identifying 'meaning units'. In one, it is a matter of carefully marking 'shifts in meaning', having placed oneself in an attitude that represents a synthesis of the phenomenological reduction and a psychological perspective. In the other, it is no more than a convenience, breaking the text into manageable pieces.

I see no way of reconciling the two explanations. If the division into meaning units is purely pragmatic, then Giorgi is quite correct to say it doesn't matter if AG and BG do it in different ways. But then what happens to the claims about 'shifts of meaning', and the specially synthesised attitude one must adopt in order to mark where these meaning shifts occur? What about the concept of meaning itself? Is it really as dispensable as the 'no theoretical weight' passage implies? Surely not, given the significance that Giorgi attaches to it elsewhere.

But then how can we explain his apparent abandonment of the idea so early in the analysis? These are questions to which we will return.

Meaning transformation

The third step in Giorgi's method requires a transformation of the meaning units into ... something else. Giorgi has various things to say about the purpose of this transformation. It involves expressing each meaning unit 'more explicitly in language revelatory of the psychological aspect of the lived-through experience with respect to the phenomenon being researched'; so that, in the example, 'one reveals as explicitly as possible the psychological sense regarding jealousy' (145). The transformation requires discipline, and its main purpose is 'to describe carefully the intuitive psychological senses that present themselves to the consciousness of the researcher' (154). This, in turn, requires 'a certain type of generalization' and a 'heightened articulation of the psychological aspect of each meaning unit' (ibid.). One does not simply attach a label to each unit; rather, one should 'exhibit, or bring forth, the psychological meaning' (ibid.). The process makes 'more manifest [the participant's] perceptions and feelings about the whole situation'. It renders 'more visible her phenomenal world' (156).

This account appears to imply that 'meaning units' have the kind of theoretical weight that, as I have just observed, Giorgi later says they do not have (179). However, for the time being, I will park that difficulty and focus on the rest. The point of the transformation is to express the 'psychological aspect' or the 'psychological sense' of the experience, in a heightened articulation. The psychological meaning of each unit is brought forth, as a result of which the participant's phenomenal world is rendered more visible. There is obviously something very important going on here, although it is surprisingly hard to say just what without using the same kind of language. It is not immediately obvious *how* to express the psychological sense, *how* to bring forth the psychological meaning, or *how* to render the subject's phenomenal world more visible. A particular kind of skilled analysis is presumably necessary, and it is reasonable to expect that Giorgi will explain exactly how that analysis is carried out.

Astonishingly, he doesn't. What he says instead is: 'It would have lengthened this section unduly to demonstrate how the transformations were worked out and such detailed work properly belongs in a workbook or practice manual' (154). Okay, well, one can respect the fact that he does not wish to extend the chapter unnecessarily; but this is surely a bit of a cop-out. The meaning transformation stage of the method is the most important of all because the 'essential structure' is based on it. So the way in which the transformations are carried out, so as to produce statements in which the 'psychological sense is brought forth', is crucial. In a chapter designed to show how the method is put into practice, Giorgi's failure to show his working is a serious omission.

On the other hand, the best way to understand how Giorgi operationalises the concept of 'bringing forth the psychological sense' of meaning units is to look closely what he (along with BG) actually does. So in the rest of this section, I will consider some examples of transformation in the hope that they will be able to throw light on the process of 'expressing the psychological aspect in a heightened articulation'.

Giorgi presents the transformation of P_1's meaning units in a matrix of 11 rows and three columns. The rows represent the 11 meaning units in P_1's story, and the columns represent the stages of the transformation from the original text (left-hand column) to final transformation (right-hand column), although sometimes the third column is blank and the second column represents the last transformation. The left-hand column, it should be noted, reproduces the original text of the story, except that the first-person text is converted into the third person.

Here is the seventh row of the matrix (Table 3.2). It is one of those in which the third column is empty, so I take it that the second column represents the final transformation of the seventh meaning unit.

Some of the changes here are unremarkable, including the employment of indirect speech ('P_1 states that…'), and the substitution of nouns for pronouns ('the situation' instead of 'it', and 'P_1's new close friend' for 'he'). But others are baffling. Consider the following transformations:

'He didn't know' → 'He was unfamiliar with'
'any of the people' → 'the people'
'in the lunch group that he went out with' → 'with whom he went out to lunch'
'that were together with them' → 'that were present at the lunch'
'that one woman' → 'that a particular woman'
'was flirting with' → 'was demonstrating a romantic interest in'
'over lunch' → [deleted]

I have absolutely no idea why the expressions in the second column express the 'psychological aspect' of the experience in a 'heightened articulation', or why they 'bring forth' the psychological meaning of each unit, or why the participant's 'phenomenal world is rendered more visible'. The changes Giorgi has made seem arbitrary, and involve either synonyms ('didn't know'/'was unfamiliar with') or minor syntactic modifications ('that he went out with'/'with whom he went out'). It seems absurd to suggest that the second expression, in each case, is psychologically more revealing than the first; and, as I have observed, Giorgi makes no attempt to explain this. Why on earth does 'a particular woman' render the

Table 3.2 AG's meaning transformation: P_1, meaning unit 7

7. Later it got worse. He didn't know any of the people in the lunch group that he went out with. P_1 found out from other friends that were together with them, that one woman in the group was flirting with him over lunch.	P_1 states that the situation got worse for her. While P_1's new close friend was unfamiliar with the people with whom he went to lunch, P_1 found out from other friends that were present at lunch that a particular woman was demonstrating romantic interest in her new close friend.

phenomenal world more visible than 'one woman'? And why is 'the people' more revelatory than 'any of the people'?

The one change that stands out a little bit from the rest is 'was demonstrating a romantic interest in' as a substitute for 'was flirting with'. Again, however, I can see no reason why the first expression 'brings forth the psychological meaning' in a way that the second does not. Indeed, in this case there is a strong argument for saying that the 'transformed' meaning subtly, but significantly, changes the sense of the original text. To 'demonstrate a romantic interest in' implies something that 'to flirt with' does not. It suggests serious hopes or intentions, whereas 'flirting' suggests more of a game. Flirting can, of course, lead to something more serious, but often it does not, and is not intended to. 'Demonstrating a romantic interest', by contrast, sounds as if it is less likely to be a game. So the shift from the left-hand column to the middle column changes the tenor of what is being said, and introduces connotations that were not in the original text. There is no indication of why Giorgi thinks this is appropriate, or why he believes that 'demonstrate a romantic interest in' expresses the 'psychological sense' better than 'to flirt with'.

Giorgi might suggest that it is inappropriate to evaluate each individual change on its own. He could, I suppose, argue that the meaning unit should be taken as a whole, not as a collection of bits. However, I don't think this is convincing. Read the two versions again, the original and the transformed. How does the transformed version 'reveal psychological meaning', holistically, in a way the original text doesn't? Is the transformed unit really more than the sum of its superficially altered parts? I can't see how. Once again, Giorgi's failure to explain 'how the transformations were worked out' makes it impossible to understand what he takes himself to be doing.

The seventh meaning unit is in no way exceptional. It's all like that. Here, for example, are some other transformations which look completely arbitrary, with the later version not expressing the 'psychological sense' any more than the earlier one (Table 3.3).

Table 3.3 AG's meaning transformations: a selection from the P_1 meaning units

each happily married to their spouses	both in happy marriages with their spouses	[omitted]
had a cold	was a bit under the weather and fatigued	< *column blank* >
she brought a snack	she provided herself with food	< *column blank* >
secretly hoping	covertly wishing	secretly entertaining the … wish
felt abandoned	felt like he deserted her	[omitted]
the same woman	the very woman	< *column blank* >
continued to flirt	continued displaying romantic behaviours	< *column blank* >

It is impossible to see why the transformation, in any of these examples, represents the 'psychological sense' in a more 'heightened articulation' than the original version. Why does 'the very woman' make P_1's 'phenomenal world' more visible than 'the same woman'? And why does 'secretly entertaining the wish' reveal more of the psychological sense than 'secretly hoping' or 'covertly wishing'? As before, the shift in meaning from 'continued to flirt' to 'continued displaying romantic behaviours' is significant but unexplained. 'Romantic behaviours' might well include kissing and touching; but the whole point of this story is that P_1's emotions were excessively aroused by mere flirting. So in this case the transformation represents a distinct change in meaning. Why? On what possible grounds? Giorgi does not explain, and the reader is left to wonder whether these shifts are completely arbitrary or, in some unfathomable way, significant.

One could ask similar questions about the move from 'felt abandoned' to 'felt like he deserted her'. In this unit, however, the third column is not left blank, but contains a further transformation. It's just that this transformation omits any reference to feeling abandoned or deserted. Why? Isn't this section of P_1's story explicitly about the sense of abandonment? Isn't this what triggers the 'emotional devastation' (to which the third column of the sixth meaning unit does refer)? How can we understand this reaction if it is not linked, psychologically, to the feeling of being abandoned? Doesn't omitting any reference to this feeling *lose* the most crucial bit of the 'psychological sense' of the original? What is Giorgi playing at here? Why does he think that omitting the 'sense of abandonment' is more revelatory, psychologically speaking, than leaving it in? We are not told.

Generalising

In some cases, of course, Giorgi would defend the transformations by pointing out that they involve 'a certain type of generalization' (154). His reasoning is that the 'psychological sense' of the meaning unit must refer to something wider than the specific circumstances portrayed in a particular story. If, for example, the transformed meaning unit included reference to 'bringing a snack', the implication would be that this had something to do with the 'structure' of jealousy, which is absurd. But why cannot the same be said of 'she provided herself with food', which is included in the final transformation? It just does not make any sense.

In another case, the generalisation (if that is what it is) loses some significant meaning, as in the case of 'felt abandoned'. Consider 'each happily married to their spouses'. This is transformed, for no apparent reason, into 'both in happy marriages with their spouses' in the second column. But the third column, which is not blank, omits all reference to the marital situation of P_1 and her friend. Why? Surely this is an important aspect of the psychology of the situation. P_1 recognises that her emotional response to feeling abandoned and to the flirting woman is excessive; and part of the reason for this, apart from the fact that the friendship is a platonic one, is that both she and the friend are happily married. If another woman was flirting with her husband, that might warrant an emotional reaction. However, in the story, the person being flirted with is someone whom she does 'not feel attracted to in a romantic way', and she frankly acknowledges the unreasonableness of her feelings. So Giorgi's transformation, possibly justified as an aspect of the generalising function, omits an important thread of meaning. How can this transformation be an expression of the 'psychological sense' in a 'heightened articulation'?

I'll return to the tension between 'generalising' and 'expressing the psychological sense' later. But it is already clear that the two objectives pull in opposite directions. Generalising involves removing features that are specific to particular cases – features such as P_1 feeling abandoned, and the fact that she and her friend are both happily married. Expressing the psychological sense in a 'heightened articulation' presumably involves identifying precisely those features. I say 'presumably', of course, because Giorgi has not explained.

Another example, from the first meaning unit (Table 3.4).

The transformations here are beyond baffling. Consider the transition from 'was with a group of people in a three-day training' to 'was with a group of people in a professional setting requiring a three-day commitment'. Relative to the generalising function, this makes sense, at least partly. 'Training' is too specific, so Giorgi substitutes 'a professional setting'. Okay, understood. (But why leave 'three-day' as it is? Isn't that overly specific as well? Why has Giorgi not replaced it with 'a few days', or a variation on that idea?) Now consider the right-hand column: 'training group that was to meet over three days'. This makes no sense. Having substituted the more general 'professional setting' for the more specific 'training', Giorgi has now, unaccountably, brought 'training' back. Why? What could possibly justify first dropping it, and then restoring it? It is impossible to tell.

There is a similar issue with gender. In the left-hand column, there are no gender terms. P_1 might be either sex, as could the friend. One might anticipate that Giorgi would preserve this gender-neutrality, as jealousy is an emotion to which both sexes are prone. The middle column, however, introduces the female pronoun, although it does not signify the sex of the close friend; whereas the right-hand column spells out the fact that P_1 is a woman, and that the friend is male. So here we have the opposite of the generalising function: with each successive transformation, the gender of the main characters becomes both more

Table 3.4 AG's meaning transformation: P_1, meaning unit 1

1 Some years ago, P_1 was with a group of people in a three-day training. P_1 had a casual friendship with some of them, and one of them P_1 had just formed a very close friendship with.	P_1 states that some years ago she was with a group of people in a professional setting requiring a three-day commitment. She states that she had a casual relationship with some of the group members, but with one of them P_1 had just formed a very close relationship.	P_1, a woman, discovered that she had formed a new, close relationship with a male member of a training group that was to meet over three days. Relationships with other members of the group were casual.

specific and more explicit. Surely Giorgi does not think that jealousy is a female emotion? But why else would he contravene his own generalisation principle in order to make the gender of each character explicit? Presumably, it is a matter of 'heightening the psychological sense', or 'rendering the participant's phenomenal world more visible'. If so, this example only serves to illustrate, once again, the inevitable tension between the 'psychological sense' objective and the generalising function. How can you meet both conditions at the same time?

Before moving on, I can't help referring to the appearance of 'discovered' in the final transformation. I just cannot see why this word is included. In the first place, P_1 says nothing about discovering anything. Second, 'discover' is a very odd word to use in this context. 'Realise' might be better. P_1 could have realised (recently?) that her friendship with the man had become a close one; but she would hardly say that she had 'discovered' this. Third, and most weirdly, the full sentence, 'P_1, a woman, discovered that she had formed a new, close relationship with a male member of a training group that was to meet over three days', might be taken to imply that she had formed the close relationship during the training event itself, or during the early stages of it. This is in contrast to the original text, which strongly implies that the friendship had been formed just before the event took place. Once again, then, Giorgi makes an inexplicable substitution, one which fits neither the generalising function nor the 'psychological sense in a heightened articulation' function. Like all his transformations – because, as I've said, it's all like this – it's puzzling, unnecessary, and completely unexplained.

The second analyst

I will compare the 'structures' of the experience of jealousy, formulated by AG and BG respectively, in a moment; but first I want to show that BG's transformations generally have the same characteristics as AG's. BG's matrix has only two columns instead of three (something AG attributes to the fact that 'AG transformed more slowly than BG'), so I will simply list a few of the changes from the original text (in the third person) to BG's single transformation (Table 3.5). The examples come from her analysis of both stories.

I don't really need to linger on these examples. They display the same unexplained characteristics as AG's own transformations: pointless synonyms ('perfect'/'flawless'), subtle but still distinct shifts in meaning ('is stunned'/'experiences disbelief'), the introduction of ambiguity ('something P_1 didn't experience very often'/'unfamiliar … to P_1'), and outright changes of sense ('luckily'/'expresses her gratitude'). The boundaries between their meaning units may be substantially different, and the actual transformations may vary; but the apparently arbitrary nature of the procedure remains the same.

Structure

According to Giorgi, the objective of a phenomenological analysis is to formulate the 'structure' of the phenomenon. This is the next stage of the process, but

Table 3.5 BG's meaning transformations: P₁ and P₂

Later it got worse	This, for P₁ a difficult situation, escalated
It was a very strange feeling, something P₁ didn't experience often.	These strong feelings seemed unfamiliar and strange to P₁.
Luckily, P₁ managed to keep her composure.	P₁ expresses her gratitude that she was able to suppress her desire to aggress against the other woman.
P₂ states that Pam is perfect.	P₂ identifies another child in her school as flawless.
Her every movement, thought and pursuit is the standard by which P₂ judges all her own.	P₂ uses the other schoolgirl as a measuring stick for judging her own worth and value.
Not friends or enemies	Neither friendly nor hostile
P₂ is stunned.	P₂ experiences disbelief.

Giorgi is predictably vague about how to get from the transformation to the structure. I will briefly review what he does say.

First we have to decide whether there is a single phenomenon being described by participants, or more than one. Giorgi suggests that the differences between the accounts can be 'intrastructural' (that is, they represent minor variations in the same phenomenon) or 'interstructural' (major differences, big enough to suggest that several phenomena have been described). But he offers no criteria on the basis of which to make this decision. It is purely impressionistic. 'The difference between the two types of structure is the type of unity that the researcher *intuits* as appropriate' (166: my italics).

Second, the structure usually consists of 'several key constituents of meaning' rather than a single idea, and the key test of the structure is 'to see if the structure collapses if a key constituent is removed' (ibid.). This involves the process of imaginative variation.

Third, the structure may include aspects of which the experiencer was unaware, even though it includes 'experiential and conscious moments seen from a psychological perspective' (ibid.).

Fourth, the psychological perspective 'implies that the lived meanings are based on an individual but get expressed eidetically, which means that they are general' (ibid.).

Fifth, the language of the transformations is sometimes carried over to the structure – but sometimes not, because the transformations are 'based upon partial analyses rather than an overview of the whole description' (167). So the writing of the structure 'takes a much more holistic perspective than the transformations themselves required' (ibid.).

None of this is particularly helpful, and Giorgi provides no guidance on how to formulate the structure, starting from the transformed meaning units. It is all a question of 'holistic perspectives' and 'what the researcher intuits as appropriate'.

The language may be congenial to people who think they know what holistic perspectives and intuition are; but, for the rest of us, it is effectively a licence to take anything that 'feels right', and call it 'analysis'. There is nothing here that serves as a check, or that provides criteria on the basis of which someone can say: 'Hang on, what justifies that?', or 'How do you know?', or 'Says who?'. Giorgi can present anything as the 'structure' of the phenomenon, and there is no basis for questioning or scepticism.

Still, let's have a look at both versions of the 'structure of jealousy', based on the two stories.

BG

Jealousy is experienced in a situation where P is not receiving sufficient attention and appreciation for herself and another person actively *robs* P of the *already lacking* attention and appreciation desired by P. Intense feelings of resentment and hostility towards the other is experienced when the other seems to take advantage of an unfair privileged position and uses this privilege to undermine P's position and P's possibility to attain the attention she seeks. P finds these negative strong emotions and physical responses uncomfortable and P intensely wishes to *hide her response*s from others.

(179)

AG

For P (an ideal), jealousy is experienced when she discovers a strong desire in herself to be the centre of attention of a significant other, or others, that is not forthcoming even though such attention would require irrational conditions. Alternatively, jealousy is experienced when P perceives that another is receiving significant attention that she wishes were being directed to her and the attention the other is receiving is experienced as a lack in her. Even though P acknowledges that a rational consideration of the situation in which jealousy occurs is understandable, the emotional investment in the desire dominates P's experience and her subjective concerns become the primary determiner of the meaning of the experience. Whether P is focusing on the attention that the other(s) are experiencing, and she is not, or focusing on the lack of proper attention that she feels is her due, her genuine feelings are not expressed to others, and the awareness of the dynamics of the situation precipitate in P feelings of physical and emotional pain. The emotional pain that P suffers also induces in P feelings of a diminished sense of self either for demanding the attention she is lacking or because aggressive and negative feelings toward the other are arising.

(167)

Giorgi's view is that these two structures 'are essentially identical even though different words are used and different dimensions of the experience are emphasised' (201). Unfortunately, I do not agree with him. The differences between AG and BG are striking, and passing them off as 'essentially identical' is an exercise in wishful thinking. Given the impressionistic nature of the whole process – the reliance on holistic perspectives and intuition – it is hardly surprising that the structures diverge as much as they do.

The structures are supposedly identical in meaning. According to Giorgi, 'an identical meaning can be expressed in multiple ways.... What matters is the meaning and not the words used to express it' (201). So he describes the disparities between AG and BG as 'linguistic differences' (ibid.). Typically, however, he provides no criteria for determining when and whether two different linguistic terms are 'essentially identical in meaning'. So the claim that the 'same meaning' underlies the two structures is something we have to take on trust; and, once again, the lack of any specifiable method gives him licence to say whatever he likes. Some of the discrepancies I note below he acknowledges himself, but he dismisses them for unconvincing reasons, which I will also evaluate.

Let me quickly run through a few of the major differences.

Alternatively

AG suggests that there are two conditions in which the structure of jealousy may be evident. He signals this by referring to the first ('Jealousy is experienced when...') and then saying: 'Alternatively, jealousy is experienced when...'. BG's structure does not reflect these two possibilities. For one researcher to point out that there are two conditions in which jealousy occurs, while the other researcher apparently fails to notice this, and instead describes just one scenario, does not inspire confidence in the 'method' they are both supposedly using.

Significant other

AG specifies that P desires to be the centre of attention of a significant other (or others), presumably thinking of P_1's close friend and P_2's schoolmates. BG mentions no such person, referring only to the attention that P does not receive. BG's account is consistent with (for example) a desire to be famous or a 'celebrity', a condition in which there is no particular 'significant other', just an undifferentiated public. There is surely a considerable difference between this kind of generic aspiration and the feelings of intense jealousy that arise in the case of husbands, wives and lovers.

Diminished sense of self

Giorgi concedes that AG emphasises a diminished sense of self, whereas BG does not.

> However, BG does say in her structure that 'P is not receiving sufficient attention and appreciation for herself' and this clearly implies that P feels that she is deserving of more attention than she is receiving and that feeling implies a certain sense of loss.
>
> (203)

This is unpersuasive. The 'identical meaning' depends on three 'implications', none of which works. First, nothing BG says implies desert. 'Not receiving sufficient attention' is consistent with simply *wanting* attention. There is no suggestion that the person in question believes she *deserves* it. Second, even if P does feel that she deserves attention, failure to get it will not necessarily be accompanied by a 'sense of loss', although it might well be accompanied by a sense of outrage, spite, or resentment. Third, a sense of loss, even if there is one, is not the same as a 'diminished sense of self'. You can experience loss without that in any way affecting your sense of self. Indeed, if you continue to believe you *deserve* whatever it is you are not getting, you cannot be said to have a 'diminished sense of self'. So the three links in Giorgi's chain of 'implication' are all very weak, and his attempt to persuade us that BG means (or, rather, 'implies') the same as AG must be judged a failure.

Implicit and explicit

'The last apparent difference,' says Giorgi, 'is that AG explicitly mentions the role of rationality and irrationality, whereas BG does not. Again, however, it is there by implication and implications are important for structures because their intent is to reduce data' (203). This doesn't make a great deal of sense. In the first place, the 'intent' of a structure is not to 'reduce data'. At least, Giorgi's earlier remarks have not mentioned this objective. Instead, he has emphasised that the purpose of a structure is to identify 'experiential and conscious moments seen from a psychological perspective', and to express these 'lived meanings' eidetically by adopting a holistic perspective. Still, let us suppose that 'to reduce data' is an additional aim.

In the second place, Giorgi appears to be claiming that, given the 'intent to reduce data', the structure will incorporate 'implications'; that is, constituents of the structure that are left implicit, instead of being explicitly referred to. But *some* formulations of the structure make these constituents explicit. In this case, for example, AG's structure does, in fact, make the 'rationality/irrationality' content explicit, even though BG's doesn't.

However, this leaves two questions hanging. First: When should a constituent of the structure be made explicit, and when can it be left implicit? (In this case, AG and BG clearly did not agree.) Second: How does a reader know when a constituent has been left implicit? If you'd only had BG's structure to go on, and not AG's, would you have realised that 'requiring irrational conditions' was an 'implication' that had been omitted in order to 'reduce the data'? (I'm reasonably sure that I wouldn't have.) Did BG think this constituent was so obvious it did not need to be spelled out? Presumably she did. But if it *is* obvious, then why did AG include it (even though doing so left 'data unreduced')? As before, Giorgi's attempt to explain away the discrepancy raises more questions than it answers.

Irrational conditions

It is not even clear what AG means when he refers to 'rational' and 'irrational'. Look again at the first sentence of his structure. 'For P … jealousy is experienced

when she discovers a strong desire in herself to be the centre of attention of a significant other, or others, that is not forthcoming even though such attention would
require irrational conditions.' What 'irrational conditions' does AG have in mind?
Why would 'irrational conditions' be required for either P_1 or P_2 to have the attention they desire?

It seems clear that AG confuses reasonableness with rationality. P_1 recognises
that her friend's decision to go out to lunch is *reasonable*, but this does not
imply – nor does she claim – that her desire for him stay with her is *irrational*.
Equally, the fact that the friend's decision to go out was reasonable does *not*
entail that for him to have stayed in with P_1 would have been irrational. Giorgi's
confusion of rational and reasonable has apparently been carried over into AG's
structure. One might perhaps agree that P_1's reaction to the flirting woman is
irrational. But this claim is different from the claim that, for her to get the attention she desires, irrational conditions would be required. In omitting 'the role of
rationality and irrationality', BG does not leave a 'constituent' of the structure
implicit. Instead, she recognises that it is irrelevant.

In any case, the 'role of rationality and irrationality' is clearly *not* implied by
BG. Giorgi argues: 'So when BG writes that "another person actually robs P of
the already lacking attention" and that "the other seems to take advantage of an
unfair privileged position", both expressions contain elements of irrational perceptions and thinking' (203). This really makes no sense at all. What is irrational
about believing that someone is taking advantage of a privileged position? The
belief may be false – it obviously *is* false in the case of P_1's story, since there is
nothing privileged about either the friend's position or the flirting woman's – but
in many cases it might be true. Either way, it is clearly not irrational. Taking
advantage is something people do, rightly or wrongly. It is not irrational to do it,
nor to believe it is being done.

On the other hand, there is certainly something rather odd about the idea that
'another person robs P of the already lacking attention'. How can anyone rob you
of something that you 'already lack'? But the irrationality in this case is BG's own.
Neither P_1 nor P_2 says anything that fits this peculiar phrase. It is something BG has
invented, adding her own imaginative interpretation to the stories, despite Giorgi's
warning that both addition and interpretation are illegitimate.

There are several other interesting and noteworthy discrepancies, but it would
be tedious to discuss them all. However, I will comment on an unexpected
remark Giorgi makes after he has tried to convince us that the two structures are
essentially identical. He says this:

> While I believe that the two structures are essentially the same, it would not
> have been a disaster if they were not. It is frequently the case that an empirical
> replication experiment does not confirm the findings of the original study.
>
> (204)

However, the analogy is unconvincing. The two structures, AG's and BG's,
are based on the *same data*. It is not as if BG has tried to replicate AG's study,

which would imply the gathering of new data, the eliciting of two new stories. The point is that AG and BG have produced structures that are significantly different, even though they claim to have analysed the same material using the same method. You can't duck this problem by saying that replications, with new material, sometimes produced different results.

The critical issue, which Giorgi does not seem to recognise, is the reliability of his 'method'. We want to know whether two or more researchers will draw the same conclusions from the same data. On this showing, they probably won't. Replication is irrelevant. Giorgi's 'method' is not really a method at all. It is rhetoric attached to what look suspiciously like arbitrary changes of wording. In which case, it is only to be expected that two different investigators, working with identical material, will produce non-identical findings.

Jealousy and envy

I suggested earlier in the chapter that P_1's story is about jealousy, in contrast to P_2's story, which is an illustration of envy. According to Tellenbach (1974) and Cobb-Stevens (2003), jealousy is a reaction to the perceived threat of loss, while envy is the desire for what someone else has.

There are several indicators of this difference between the two. First, jealousy is associated with a desire for exclusivity: A wants exclusive rights to a relationship with C, and sees B as threatening those rights. In contrast, envy is not a desire to possess something exclusively. It is not a zero-sum game. If A envies B his wealth, she doesn't necessarily want more money than B, nor does she necessarily wish to deprive B of his riches. She merely wants to be equally wealthy.

Second, the object of desire is different. In the case of envy, A may covet B's wealth, success, character, situation, fame, various goods, and so on. In cases of jealousy, the object of desire is a person. A wants to preserve her relationship with C, and is jealous of anybody (B) who poses a threat to that relationship.

Third, jealousy is related to fear. It is part of the 'fear-of-loss' family. Envy, in contrast, is more closely related to greed, and is part of the 'desire' family.

In summary, jealousy is a three-term relation in which A wants exclusive rights to another person, C, and fears B as a threat. Envy is a two-term relation in which A is non-exclusively greedy for the non-personal goods possessed by B.

However, it is true that 'jealous' is often used as a synonym of 'envious', as well as in the sense just defined. I might say that I am jealous of Gerald's success, meaning that I envy him; but this is different from the situation in which charming, good-looking Alfred dancing with my wife makes me jealous. In the first case, 'jealousy' is a rough equivalent of 'envy'; in the second case, it is specific to relationship rivalry. The 'envy' sense is not illegitimate; but we need to bear in mind that it is distinct from the fear-of-loss, relationship sense.

This brings us back to an important question that came up earlier in the chapter: how do we pick out a 'phenomenon'? On what basis do we draw a boundary round the proposed subject of study? How do we distinguish between the phenomenon of interest and an 'adjacent' phenomenon, and on what criteria?

These are questions to which, as I noted earlier, Giorgi provides no answer. In the case of the 'jealousy' example, the question becomes: are jealousy and envy just aspects of the same phenomenon? Or are they different phenomena? And on what basis do we decide?

My own view will be evident by now. 'Jealousy' is a word with more than one use. The dictionary (the OED in this case) identifies six different senses. I have distinguished between two of them, one being the fear-of-loss sense, and the other being broadly synonymous with 'envy'. It seems likely that, in the workshop, P_1 interpreted 'jealousy' in its fear-of-loss sense, whereas P_2 interpreted it in its synonymous-with-envy sense. Giorgi does not appear to have considered this possibility. Instead, he tries to formulate a single 'structure', even though two different phenomena have been described.

It is not possible to specify an object of study simply by adopting a word, as if words and 'phenomena' corresponded in simple one-to-one relations (for every word, a phenomenon; for every phenomenon, a word). The only way to do it, as I shall argue in Chapter 7, is to make use of prior scientific knowledge, including prior psychological knowledge. For the most part, this will be knowledge of cause and effect.

Lived confusedly

Towards the end of his chapter on jealousy, Giorgi refers briefly to the distinction made by Tellenbach (1974) and Cobb-Stevens (2003). He is unimpressed. 'While these distinctions make sense formally and in the abstract, the data show that the two emotions can be lived confusedly in one situation' (204).

But this is not the situation at all. Consider another of his remarks: 'I asked for descriptions of jealousy, and according to the above definitions, got envy as well' (204). This is precisely the problem: 'I asked for descriptions of jealousy'. If you believe in the 'one word, one phenomenon' theory, then 'asking for descriptions of jealousy' looks like an unambiguous request. However, 'jealousy', as I have suggested, has a number of different senses, including the two specified above. If participants are asked to describe 'jealousy', with no further explanation of what is required, there is nothing to stop them interpreting that word in different ways (as P_1 and P_2 appear to have done). If the participants' choice is not in some way policed, the result will be a rag-bag of interpretation, with no guarantee that the situations described have much in common at all.

The problem is not that two different emotions can be 'lived confusedly in one situation'. It is rather that a single emotion can be given either of two different labels, and that two different emotions can be given the same label. *Either* you covet someone else's goods and status, *or* you fear that another person might deprive you of the love of a significant other. The trouble is that both of these situations can be described with an ambiguous word: 'jealousy'. So if there is 'confusion' in any of this, it lies in Giorgi's failure to see that 'jealousy' is an ambiguous term, and that it cannot be identified with a single 'phenomenon'.

Attention and resentment

Earlier, I focused on the differences between AG's and BG's structures, emphasising that the 'method' that Giorgi recommends produces different results.
However, it is worth considering the similarities too, because they reveal the
degree of confusion from which Giorgi and his wife both suffer. Trying to find
an analysis that reduces P_1's jealousy and P_2's envy to a common denominator,
they produce a convoluted account that does not even reflect the two stories.
Consider BG's structure, for example:

> Jealousy is experienced in a situation where P is not receiving sufficient
> attention and appreciation for herself and another person actively *robs* P of
> the *already lacking* attention and appreciation desired by P.

This may fit P_2's story, if we ignore the odd idea that one can be robbed of what
one lacks, but to what extent does it capture P_1's? In her story, P_1 does not
receive 'sufficient attention and appreciation' from the 'new close friend'. So
far, so good. But in what sense does the flirtatious woman rob P_1 of the close
friend's attention? According to the story, not at all. It is the flirtatious woman
who is paying attention to the close friend, not the other way round. 'One woman
in the group was flirting with him.... When we were all back in the group
together, she continued to flirt with him. He looked at her in amazement, as did
everyone.' There is no suggestion, anywhere in the story, that the friend flirted
back. So in what sense is the flirtatious woman robbing P_1 of the attention she
desires? This is, transparently, an attempt to get P_1's story to conform to the template of P_2's. The rest of BG's structure makes the same error:

> Intense feelings of resentment and hostility towards the other is experienced
> when the other seems to take advantage of an unfair privileged position and
> uses this privilege to undermine P's position and P's possibility to attain the
> attention she seeks.

The flirtatious woman may have *wished* to 'undermine P_1's position', but there
is no indication that she succeeded. Moreover, it should be noted that, in P_2's
story, resentment is directed towards the *receiver* of attention. In P_1's, however,
the resentment is directed towards the *giver* of attention (that is, the flirt).

If we see BG's structure as an attempt to construe a story of envy and a story
of jealousy as essentially the same, we can finally understand the strange idea
that P is robbed of 'already lacking attention'. The 'already lacking' fits P_1's
account, because P_1 did not receive her friend's attention over lunch. But the
'being robbed' clearly fits P_2's story (and does not fit P_1's), because P_2 thinks
that Pam is depriving her of attention that, in a fairer world, would come to her.
So take the 'already lacking' from P_1's story, and the 'being robbed' from P_2's
... and splice them together. 'Already lacking' makes sense in P_1's story, and
'being robbed' makes sense in P_2's. But they make no sense whatever when

combined in the odd phrase 'actively *robs* P of the *already lacking* attention and appreciation desired by P'.

It is the attempt to make the two stories fit the same template, to pretend that the two phenomena are the same, that creates this peculiar impossibility.

Imaginative variation

The test of an essential structure, according to Giorgi, is to see whether it 'collapses if a key constituent is removed' (166). This test requires the use of imaginative variation, in which thought experiments – the removal of candidate 'key constituents' – are carried out. If the structure 'collapses' when the constituent in question is removed, then the constituent is essential. If it doesn't, then it isn't. 'The attainment of the structure is not based on facts alone, but also on eidetic intuitions' (199).

Giorgi provides an example (197). It involves the imaginative removal of specific constituents from P_2's story, including the pretty young girl and the horse. The removal of these details does not cause the structure to collapse, so Giorgi correctly infers that not all cases of 'jealousy' (or envy) include details of this kind.

However, it is difficult to understand why other constituents are included in AG's structure because, on the face of it, they are no more essential to the phenomenon 'jealousy' than pretty young girls and horses. Take the reference to 'physical and emotional pain', for example. Is physical pain an essential constituent of jealousy? It is interesting that BG doesn't mention it. Her structure includes 'negative strong emotions and physical responses'; but she does not refer to 'pain' (and pain is obviously much more specific than 'physical response', which might be nausea, crawling skin, blushing, sweating, and so on).

This is another discrepancy between AG and BG. Here, however, I am more interested in the 'collapsing structure' test of imaginative variation. It would appear that 'physical pain' passes AG's version of the test – it must be an essential constituent, so is included in the structure – but not BG's. And since Giorgi does not provide criteria, it is impossible to decide whose imaginative variation 'thought experiment' is correct. Did the structure collapse for AG, but remain intact for BG, when physical pain was removed? Presumably. But then what kind of a test is this, if it has a different outcome for different researchers?

There are other examples of constituents that are included in the structures, but that look as if they would not precipitate collapse if they were to be removed. The diminished sense of self (not included in BG's structure) is one we have discussed already, along with 'irrational conditions'. But one constituent retained by both AG and BG is P-hiding-her-feelings. She 'intensely wishes to hide her responses from others' (BG); 'her genuine feelings are not expressed to others' (AG). But on the face of it, this is not an essential characteristic of jealousy (or indeed envy). There are surely plenty of cases in which the jealous/envious person's feelings are visible, and when he or she does not bother to conceal them. To that extent, then, the structure does not collapse when this constituent is removed.

Giorgi might suggest that 'hiding one's feelings' is essential to the structure of jealousy-as-experienced-by-P_1-and-P_2. But, if that's right, why bother with imaginative variation in the first place? The point of the procedure was to determine the effect of removing certain features of the original stories in order to identify the essential structure of *jealousy*, not the essential structure of *two-particular-accounts-of-jealousy*. If the removal of anything common to both stories inevitably implies the collapse of the essential structure, the procedure is pointless. As in previous examples, it is the inconsistency of Giorgi's 'method', coupled with his failure to explain or justify any of the details, which is bewildering.

Meaning unexplained

Giorgi's phenomenological method, illustrated by the extended example of jealousy, turns out to be a mirage. Every example of meaning attribution in the various stages of analysis – the creation of meaning units, the transformations, the development of a structure – appears to be based on nothing more than arbitrary decisions made by AG and BG. Giorgi has insufficient space, so he claims, to 'demonstrate how the transformations were worked out'. But the truth is that he explains hardly any of the methodological decisions arising out of the creation of meaning units, meaning transformation, and the formulation of essential structures; and even some of the explanations he does give don't make much sense.

Throughout the analysis, Giorgi appeals to his (and his wife's) intuitions about 'meaning'. He claims that meaning-unit boundaries are identified whenever a 'shift in meaning' takes place in the participant's story (although later he suggests that meaning units are just a convenient way of breaking the story into smaller pieces; they have no theoretical weight). The point of the transformations is to 'exhibit, or bring forth, the psychological meaning of what was said', with 'heightened articulation'. And the finished structure consists of 'key constituent meanings', which survive the test of 'structural collapse'. So the identification, transformation and testing of meaning define Giorgi's whole enterprise. On this showing, 'meaning' is the most important concept in phenomenology. But Giorgi never explains what he means by it, and never subjects it to any form of analysis.

But an analysis of some kind is clearly necessary. A close examination of the 'jealousy' example shows that, at every stage, 'meaning' is an indeterminate and highly malleable idea. The boundaries between the meaning units are identified in different ways by the two researchers; but this apparently 'doesn't matter'. The psychological meaning, which is the point of the transformations, turns out to be whatever Giorgi says it is, since there is no way to account for the arbitrary substitutions, the sudden additions, the random synonyms, the unexplained interpretations, the surprising confusions, or the concepts seemingly picked out of the air. The essential structures produced by AG and BG have 'identical meanings', even though they are radically different. Some of the 'constituent meanings' of jealousy pass the 'collapse of structure' test; others don't. And the semantic boundaries between different meanings of 'jealousy' are never defined, permitting Giorgi to confuse jealousy with envy (though he imagines that the confusion is the result of the two emotions being 'lived confusedly in one situation').

In Chapter 5, I will undertake my own analysis of the words 'means' and 'meaning'. First, however, I want to look at the work of another influential methodologist, Max van Manen, and determine whether his analytical procedures are any clearer, and any more subject to identifiable criteria, than Giorgi's.

Note

1 Giorgi accepts that there is a difference between PP and PQR ('scientific phenomenology'), but he nevertheless claims 'phenomenological status' for his method. However, given that he reverses and/or dismantles every significant feature of Husserl's phenomenology, it is difficult to see how he can justify awarding 'phenomenological status' to 'scientific phenomenology'. Consider the systematic differences. Husserl: present-tense data derived from outside the natural attitude by a lone philosopher who, having performed the epoché, abstains from all judgment and positing, and describes (in an intrinsically error-free way) the abstracted structures of experience-in-general. Giorgi's scientific phenomenology: past-tense accounts (in which error is always possible) of specific, concrete experiences provided by several respondents who are unfamiliar with phenomenology, and who speak from inside the judgement-laden natural attitude of everyday awareness. Since nothing of Husserl remains in 'scientific phenomenology', how can Giorgi grant it 'phenomenological status'?

References

Cobb-Stevens R. (2003) 'Husserl's fifth logical investigation', in D. O. Dahlstrom (ed.) *Husserl's Logical Investigations*. Dordrecht: Kluwer Academic, pp. 95–107.

Giorgi A. (2009) *The Descriptive Phenomenological Method in Psychology: A Modified Husserlian Approach*. Pittsburgh: Duquesne University Press.

Holland A. C. and Kensinger E. A. (2010) 'Emotion and autobiographical memory', *Physics of Life Reviews*, 7(1), pp. 88–131.

Kassin S. M., Tubb V. A., Hosch H. M. and Memon A. (2001) 'On the "general acceptance" of eyewitness testimony research', *American Psychologist*, 56(5), pp. 405–416.

Loftus E. F. (1979) *Eyewitness Testimony*. Cambridge, MA: Harvard University Press.

Schacter D. L. and Addis D. R. (2007) 'The ghosts of past and future: a memory that works by piecing together bits of the past may be better suited to simulating future events than one that is a store of perfect records', *Nature*, 445(7123), p. 27.

Tellenbach H. (1974) 'On the nature of jealousy', *Journal of Phenomenological Psychology*, 4(2), pp. 461–468.

4   Max van Manen

Being left or abandoned

Max van Manen is perhaps the most frequently cited methodological authority in the PQR literature. In a number of respects, he and Giorgi are very different writers. Stylistically, they vary enormously. Giorgi is clear but prosaic; van Manen's writing is much flashier, but it is not always obvious what he means. From a philosophical point of view, Giorgi's main point of reference is the descriptive phenomenology associated with Husserl; van Manen draws on both descriptive and interpretive traditions. Van Manen's most cited book (1990) is less technical than Giorgi's; but Giorgi tries harder (though unsuccessfully) to present a 'method'. Indeed, van Manen rejects the idea of method, and substitutes something he calls a 'methodos'.

Each of these differences is worth considering more closely. On the one hand, van Manen's style makes his work difficult to pin down. On the other, his attempt to meld together the descriptive and interpretive threads in the phenomenological tradition is responsible for a series of (what appear to be) anomalies in his account of meaning attribution.

Style

Van Manen's writing is full of bold gestures, fuzzy ideas, and unargued-for claims. Examples of these claims include: 'research is a caring act'; 'we can only understand something or someone for whom we care'; 'love is foundational for all knowing of human existence'; 'phenomenology, not unlike poetry, is a poetising project'; and 'we must engage language in a primal incantation or poetising which harkens back to the silence from which the words emanate' (van Manen 1990: 5–13). Anyone looking for a rigorously analytic textbook should approach with caution.

After an opening in which love is declared to be foundational for human knowing, it is inevitable that 'mystery' will turn up eventually; and it does, in a discussion of parenting. But it is a mystery that can, in a certain, non-standard, highly convoluted sense, be *known*.

> The mystery of parenting is knowable.... Parenting is an utter mystery, yet knowable. The project of a phenomenology of parenting is, therefore, not to

translate (reduce) the primordial relationship of parenting into clearly defined concepts so as to dispel its mystery, but rather the object is to bring the mystery more fully into our presence.

(Van Manen 1990: 50)

It is an idea to which van Manen returns on several occasions. Later, while developing the concept of a 'theme', he says: 'No thematic formulation can completely unlock the deep meaning, the full mystery, the enigmatic aspects of the experiential meaning of a notion' (88); 'no conceptual formulation or single statement can possibly capture the full mystery' (92).

In other words, the phenomenologist can come to 'know' the phenomenon she has studied, but not by conceptualising it. The 'full mystery' of the phenomenon will remain locked away, and the mystery will be *utter*. But it can be brought into her 'presence'. If the alarm bells weren't ringing before, they should be now.

In a different context, these references to mystery, and the claim that 'there is always an element of the ineffable to life' (16), might be dismissed as a bit of purple prose that needn't be taken too seriously. But van Manen's work has influenced a great deal of research, in nursing as well as in education, and it is not self-evident that the 'mysterious' and the 'ineffable' are useful concepts in health care. Nor is it obvious that van Manen's style, with its abstruse metaphors and endemic imprecision, is an adequate model for the painstaking analysis and critical distinctions that good research in any discipline requires.

Van Manen does appear to have wondered about this himself: 'Some argue that phenomenology has no practical value because "you cannot do anything with phenomenological knowledge"' (45). But he swiftly rejects this thought. 'The more important question is not: Can we do something with phenomenology? Rather, we should wonder: Can phenomenology, if we concern ourselves deeply with it, do something with us?' (ibid.). Seriously, that's what he says. But he doesn't attempt to justify the assertion that the second question is 'more important', or to explain what 'phenomenology doing something with us' would look like. The rhetorical effect turns on the reader being impressed by an incomprehensible idea.

It is difficult to engage critically with writing like this, because it avoids committing itself to anything definite. In fact, it makes a virtue of fuzziness. Van Manen himself concedes that 'human science is often accused of yielding texts that are vague, imprecise, inexact, non-rigorous, or ambiguous'; and he recognises that 'scholars such as Merleau-Ponty, Heidegger, Levinas, or Derrida employ seemingly evasive or even poetic writing styles and ways of saying things that seem elusive'. But his riposte is:

> It may be that such styles and means of expression are the concomitants of a more richly embodied notion of human rationality.... Furthermore, we should acknowledge that human science operates with its own criteria for precision, exactness and rigor.

(17)

This comes close to claiming that 'evasive' is the new rational, and 'elusive' is the new precise. It also suggests that readers of his book will not find their way cluttered with anything as vulgar – as not-richly-rational – as precise claims and clear arguments.

Philosophical anomalies

There are several anomalies in van Manen's book, arising out of his project to combine the descriptive and interpretive traditions in phenomenology. These anomalies all take the same form: a technical term is used in inconsistent ways, or contradictory statements are made about a key phenomenological idea. I should perhaps say 'apparently inconsistent' and 'apparently contradictory'; but van Manen's style is so breathless that he never pauses to suggest: 'Okay, that might sound as if it is inconsistent with the claim I made on the previous page; but here's why it isn't…'. So the reader must try to reconcile the conflicting passages without any help from the author. I will consider a couple of examples.

Non-reflective consciousness

Van Manen oscillates between two accounts of what is studied by phenomenologists. The first account is that phenomenology investigates 'experience as we live it rather than as we conceptualize it' (30). This as-we-live-it experience occurs in a 'non-thematic, non-reflective type of consciousness', and van Manen references Merleau-Ponty in claiming that the aim of phenomenology is to 're-achieve a direct and primitive contact with the world' (38, citing Merleau-Ponty 1962 [1945]: vii), the world as it is immediately experienced. 'Basic things about our lifeworld … are preverbal and therefore hard to describe' (18); and phenomenology differs from other sciences in that it tries to 'gain insightful descriptions of the way we experience the world pre-reflectively, without taxonomizing, classifying or abstracting' (9). This sounds as if 'pre-verbal' and 'non-reflective' amount to the same thing; and van Manen seems to confirm this by suggesting that 'biking consciousness', as an example of pre-reflective consciousness, is not a consciousness *of* biking (38). The task of phenomenology, on this account, appears to be the difficult one of finding words to describe pre-verbal, pre-conceptual, pre-classified experiences.

The second account appears to be the complete opposite. Citing 'postmodernism, deconstructionism, and other language-oriented human science approaches', van Manen observes that 'lived experience is soaked through with language' (38). 'Human experience is only possible because we have language', and 'lived experience itself seems to have a linguistic structure' (39).

How is this possible? Experience-as-we-live-it was initially contrasted with as-we-conceptualize-it. It was supposed to be non-reflective, non-thematic; and at least some basic aspects of it were supposed to be preverbal. Now, suddenly, lived experience is *soaked through* with language; more, it has a linguistic structure. But how can it be soaked in language and remain at the same time, preverbal, non-reflective, and non-conceptualised? Is there a form of language that does not involve concepts, or that can be described as 'preverbal'? Surely, if lived experience has a linguistic structure, it embodies concepts, taxonomies and classification. Can anything be linguistic – sodden with language – and at the same time a preverbal, non-classifying, concept-free zone?

This ambiguity about experience is a result of van Manen's eclecticism, his willingness to embrace both descriptive phenomenology and interpretivism/ hermeneutics. The first is associated, according to van Manen, with preverbal, non-reflective consciousness, the second with language-soaked lived experience. I am prepared to believe that the two apparently incompatible accounts can be reconciled. It's just that van Manen provides no clues as to how this rapprochement can be effected.

Culture and history

Van Manen suggests that phenomenology 'does not aim to explicate meanings specific to particular cultures ... [or] to historical periods' (11). But on the next page, he argues that phenomenological research must take into account 'the socio-cultural and historical traditions that have given meaning to our ways of being in the world', and proposes that one phenomenology project might be to 'understand what it means to be a woman in our present age' (12). Later, he argues that 'even themes that would appear to be essential meanings are often historically and culturally determined or shaped' (106).

So which is it? Is phenomenology the study of non-historical, non-cultural meaning, the meaning-of-the-phenomenon stripped of historical and cultural accoutrements? Or is it the study of meanings 'gifted' by socio-cultural and historical traditions? Again, the first is associated with descriptive phenomenology, the second with phenomenological hermeneutics. Van Manen's inconsistencies are the result of his wish to draw on a combination of both types.

Despite the challenges posed both by his style and his best-of-both-worlds philosophy, I'll make a stab at evaluating van Manen's work in this chapter. I will examine two of his examples and, as with Giorgi, try to determine how he gets from text to meaning. First, however, I think it is necessary to discuss what he actually says about method.

Method and morality

Giorgi presents a method based on 'scientific phenomenology'. Van Manen, in contrast, rejects the idea of a phenomenological method altogether. At least, he in-a-manner-of-speaking rejects it.

> So in a serious sense there is not really a 'method' understood as a set of investigative procedures that one can master relatively quickly. Indeed it has been said that *the method of phenomenology and hermeneutics is that there is no method!*
>
> (29–30: italics original)

You can hear the 'but' coming. 'And yet, it is not entirely wrong to say that phenomenology and hermeneutics as described here definitely have a certain *methodos* – a way'.

The *methodos* does not involve 'fixed signposts' (29): it is not a recipe, and it can't be followed in a sequence of steps. Rather, it is embodied in a tradition. 'While it is true that the method of phenomenology is that there is no method, yet there is a tradition', and this tradition constitutes the 'methodological ground for present human science research' (30). But the tradition is not prescriptive: phenomenological inquiry neither 'rejects or ignores this tradition, nor slavishly follows or kneels in front of it' (ibid.).

This sounds rather grand, but it doesn't have much informative content. There is no method, but there is a *methodos*. The tradition embodying the *methodos* is the 'methodological ground' of research, but it is not to be followed slavishly; nor should it be ignored. Van Manen tells us that the tradition incorporates 'a body of knowledge and insights', together with a 'history of lives of thinkers and authors' that can be 'taken as an example'. But he does not specify the body of knowledge (or provide any examples of it); and he does not say in what respect certain unnamed thinkers had 'lives' that can be taken as 'an example'. However, even if we knew who these thinkers were, and which aspects of their lives could be taken as an example, we would still have no idea what *not* following their example 'slavishly' would involve (or not involve, as the case may be).

The problem with talk about a *methodos*, an unspecified, non-prescriptive 'way', is that it is consistent with there being no constraints on enquiry at all. What prevents it becoming a blank cheque, a licence to say whatever you find congenial? Can anyone ask: 'How do you know?', or say: 'I think you've got that wrong.'? Are there any checks, any benchmarks, any criteria by which the phenomenologist's work can be judged? Or is the *methodos* just an exercise in wheeling out preferred 'meanings', with the occasional reassuring reference to 'the history of lives of thinkers'? If it isn't an arbitrary exercise, how do we know it isn't? How can van Manen, or anyone else, convince us that his analysis is not merely a reflection of his own priorities and preferences?

This worry is intensified by what van Manen says about interpretation. Like all phenomenology writers, he proposes to tell us the meaning of an experience, or a phenomenon, or a text. However, 'expressing the fundamental or overall meaning of a text is a judgment call' (94). Furthermore, 'different readers might discern different fundamental meaning. And it does not make one interpretation necessarily more true than another' (ibid.). Interpretation is not 'rule-bound', but rather 'a free act of "seeing" meaning' (79). It follows that 'a phenomenological description is always *one* interpretation, and no single interpretation of human experience will ever exhaust the possibility of yet another complementary, or even potentially *richer* or *deeper* description' (31).

The idea that different interpretations of the same material are equally true, that one is not necessarily more true than another, is probably more familiar now than it was in 1990. It presumably applies even when the different interpretations are inconsistent with each other – for example, if one of them implies S, while another implies the opposite, not-S. In a situation of that kind, formal logic would say that at least one of them must be false, because S and the opposite-of-S cannot both be true. However, we are dealing with *interpretation* here, so perhaps logic is not relevant. In any case, van Manen includes the word 'complementary', and suggests that new interpretations might be 'richer' or 'deeper'. So possibly he thinks that incompatible, non-complementary interpretations never arise.

Still, without criteria for determining when one interpretation is indeed richer or deeper than another, we are not much further forward. For example, why can't I just claim that my interpretation is 'deeper' than van Manen's, or 'richer', or in some other way 'better', even if it is not more true? Is there any way in which the matter can be adjudicated? Is there any means of confirming that my interpretation *is* 'deeper' or 'richer' than his? To repeat the earlier question, what is it that prevents 'interpreting overall meaning' from becoming a matter of personal preference?

I think van Manen has two answers to this question. Here is one of them: 'Perhaps the best answer to the question of what is involved in a hermeneutic phenomenological human science research method is "scholarship!"' (29). He continues: 'A human science researcher is a scholar: a sensitive observer of the subtleties of everyday life, and an avid reader of relevant texts'. In other words, we have to take it on trust. There are *no* constraints, checks, criteria, or benchmarks. There are no methods for distilling meaning, no procedures for identifying error. It all comes down to one idea. Trust me, I'm a scholar.

That is the first answer to the 'Isn't it just arbitrary?' question. The second provides a criterion for what counts as a good phenomenological description. 'Buytendijk once referred to the "phenomenological nod" as a way of indicating that a good phenomenological description is something that we can nod to, recognising it as an experience that we have had or could have had' (27). Van Manen clearly endorses this idea, and continues: 'A good phenomenological description ... is validated by lived experience' (ibid.).

The 'phenomenological nod' has proved a popular notion, and turns up in research textbooks (Munhall 1994). It is also cited in recent PQR studies (Burhans and Alligood 2010; Hughes *et al.* 2010). However, its implications are deeply disturbing. A 'good' phenomenological description is one that people assent to? Really? Doesn't that mean that research on 'meaning' can never produce surprising results? If the test of a good study is that the reader says 'Yes, of course, that's right!', then phenomenology can never come up with a conclusion that prompts the reader to say, instead: 'Gosh, that's a shock', or 'That's hard to believe', or 'Let me just go over that again, because the findings are counterintuitive, and I want to check the methodological basis for them'. If the 'phenomenological nod' really is the test of a good study, then phenomenology can never tell us anything we didn't already know, or aren't willing to accept more or less instantly. In which case, what's the point of it?

There is a strand in van Manen's thinking that is in tension with phenomenological nods and the idea that one interpretation is no more true than another. This is the claim that phenomenological description has moral importance.

In phenomenological research description carries a moral force. If to be a father means to take active responsibility for a child's growth, then it is possible to say of actual cases that this or that is no way to be a father!'

(12)

In other words, if phenomenology indicates that being a father means doing X and being Y, then any male parent not doing X or being Y is not a proper father; and the implication is that this counts as a moral deficit. We can say that he *ought* to do X and be Y, on the grounds that this is what being a father *means*.

Any claim about the world that supports this kind of moral judgment had better be true. Suppose we say:

S is true, therefore you ought to do X.

In this example, the moral force of that judgment hangs precisely on S being true. It would be far less persuasive to say:

My interpretation is S, therefore you ought to do X. However, S is no more true than not-S.

So van Manen's willingness to put this sort of moral weight on phenomenological conclusions about 'meaning' does not sit comfortably with his claim that 'a phenomenological description is always *one* interpretation, and no single interpretation of human experience will ever exhaust' the possibilities.

On the other hand, combining the 'moral force' with the 'phenomenological nod' is quite scary. Think about it. Some ill-defined community gives the nod to an account of what it 'means' to be a father, or what it 'means to be a woman in our present age'. On the basis of this assent, they lay down the law about what fathers should do, and what women shouldn't do, because the 'meaning' has 'moral force'. Even more topically, consider the claim that the 'meaning of marriage' is the union of one man and one woman. If this claim gets the phenomenological nod, the opposition to same-sex marriage has moral force. And, according to van Manen, there is no court of appeal beyond that nod. This is an inherently conservative position, with no independent point of reference from which that-just-seems-right-to-me conclusions can be challenged.

According to Sparrow (2014), quoted in Chapter 2, 'a method is supposed to rein in spurious conjecture and speculative impulses' (5). However, van Manen rejects the idea of a method. He prefers tradition, and the not-slavish following of exemplary thinkers. This, as I have argued, is an intrinsically conservative position. But the key methodological question is: In the absence of a *method* that gets you from text to meaning, how does van Manen propose to elucidate meaning? What form do his meaning attributions take? What is it that occupies the slot vacated by method? It is all very well talking about a methodos, tradition and example, but the question of the 'How-does-he-do-it-in-a-particular-case?' detail still has to be answered.

In the rest of this chapter, I consider two of van Manen's examples. I argue that meaning attribution in these examples is not based on 'a reading from within the text itself', but on moral judgments of his own. Specifically, he appears to have some well-defined views about parenting; and, coincidentally, it turns out that these views are vindicated by his phenomenological studies of what parenting *means*.

Being left, being abandoned

In Chapter 3, I argued that Giorgi fails to explain how he draws the boundary between 'phenomena'. He provides no guidance on how to pick out a particular phenomenon for study, or how to determine where one phenomenon stops and another starts. In his analysis of jealousy, it became apparent that he confuses jealousy with envy, that his 'structure' includes other emotions, not necessarily related to jealousy, and that several components of the 'essence' are not essential.

The same problem occurs in van Manen's examples, and particularly in the analysis of a phenomenon he calls 'feeling left or abandoned'. The data for this example consists of a series of 12 descriptions, six of which are overtly fictional (*Hansel and Gretel*; *Sophie's Choice;* a short story by Anna Blaman; Truffaut's *Small Change;* Marilynne Robinson's novel, *Housekeeping;* and *Disobedience*, a poem by A. A. Milne). Other than these six, it is not clear where the descriptions come from.

The descriptions are extremely varied. A boy who is left at home with a babysitter when his parents go to a movie; a boy who is left alone at home while his parents go out for a walk; parents who leave their 11-year-old daughter at home when they go out to Sunday brunch; a father dropping his children off at school; a child who is afraid that his mother will never return when she goes 'down to the end of town' without him; a father who takes his daughter to day care, where she spends seven or eight hours a day; a boy who spends ten hours a day in a day-care centre, and who seems unresponsive when the assistant says goodbye; a six-year-old boy who is left at home with his sister and a nanny when his parents go on holiday; a mother who, following a divorce, leaves the family home and her four-year-old son, never to return; a girl whose only parent, her mother, commits suicide; a mother forced by the Nazis to choose which child to leave behind; a brother and sister who are left to fend for themselves in the forest, and who are subsequently threatened by a cannibalistic witch (80–85).

The implication is that these are all examples of the same phenomenon, 'feeling left or abandoned'. But on what basis does van Manen lump together a father dropping his children off at school, and a woman abandoning her son after a divorce? Or a boy left at home with a babysitter when his parents go out for the evening, and a girl whose single-parent mother commits suicide? Or a father who takes his daughter to day care, and parents who abandon their children in a forest? On what grounds does he suppose that leaving your children – temporarily, for a short period – in the care of another responsible person is the 'same phenomenon' as absenting yourself from them *permanently*, without making any provision for their safety or welfare?

At no point does van Manen offer a justification for this procedure. He simply classifies dropping off a child at school as the *same thing* as a single parent committing suicide, a divorced mother leaving her son for ever, and a woman forced to leave one of her two children in a Nazi concentration camp.

An understandable reaction to this classification is that it is absurd. How can these possibly be regarded as the 'same phenomenon'? It is like suggesting that a walk down to the local chemist and flying to New Zealand are the same thing because they can both be classified as 'leaving the house'; or that poisoning somebody and treating them for infection with antibiotics are the same phenomenon because they both involve administering chemicals. This is the same problem that I drew attention to before: how general, or how specific, does the specification of a 'phenomenon' have to be? By what criteria do we determine where the boundaries between phenomena are? Is 'walking to the local shops' a different phenomenon from 'flying to New Zealand'? Or are they instances of the same phenomenon, 'leaving the house'? Is 'being dropped off at school for the day' a different phenomenon from 'being permanently abandoned by a single-parent mother'? Or are they examples of the same phenomenon, 'being left or abandoned'? In either case, whatever answer is proposed, how do we know? How can we discriminate? What is the *basis* for this methodological classification-decision?

Van Manen obviously believes that 'being left or abandoned' is a phenomenon that encompasses both the child being dropped off at school and the single-parent mother committing suicide. But he makes no attempt to explain why, nor does he provide even a sketchy discussion of the issues involved. There is, however, a hint of his thinking in the discussion that precedes the 12 descriptions. 'This feeling of being left is especially common with young children. What does a parent do with such situations? It depends on how the parent understands the child's experience of feeling left or abandoned' (80). So perhaps van Manen assumes that the *child's experience* is the same, whatever the actual circumstances. There is a 'feeling of being left or abandoned' that children experience, and that is common to the different descriptions, irrespective of whether the child is left with the babysitter for the evening, or is permanently abandoned by his divorced mother. Perhaps it is this common thread that justifies all 12 scenarios being classified as one phenomenon, 'being left or abandoned'.

Unfortunately, there are two problems with this line of thought. The first is that it is circular. How does van Manen know that the child's experience is the same *before* he carries out the study? Isn't the whole point of a phenomenological study to *determine* what the experience of the 'phenomenon' is like? So the criterion for picking out the 'phenomenon' in the first place must be independent of the conclusions about the experience we propose to study. Van Manen's logic, on this account, would be: 'I am going to study people's experience of situations A, B and C (which I will classify as the single phenomenon, X, because the experiences of A, B and C are the same)'. If that is right, van

Manen already knows what his conclusion will be, and presupposes it in the very act of defining the 'phenomenon'.

The second problem is that the data in this example, the 12 descriptions, do not support the claim that children's experience of 'being left and abandoned' is the same. In one case, for example, David and his brother react quite differently to being left with the babysitter for the evening. David wants to know how long his parents will be, and says: 'Come straight back home, okay?'; his brother 'hardly takes notice that his parents are leaving' (81). Likewise, the two siblings in another description have quite disparate reactions. Tommy rushes off to the playground when he is dropped off at school, but his sister Julie wants to know where her parents will be during the day, and quizzes her father in order to find out (81–82). The girl left behind during Sunday lunch (in Truffaut's film) is triumphant when she attracts the attention of neighbours, who hoist a generously filled food basket up to the third-story window (83–84). Martin Buber, abandoned by his divorced mother, initially expected her to return; but, a year later, he came to understand that she never would, and 'it stayed with me and each year it affixed itself more deeply to my heart' (84). For Ruth (in the novel by Marilynne Robinson), whose single parent mother commits suicide, 'life becomes one long endless waiting' (85). And so on.

Where, in any of this, is the evidence that the children's experience of 'being left or abandoned' is the same? Where is the justification for claiming that Tommy's experience of being dropped off at school and Buber's experience of being abandoned by his mother are the 'same phenomenon'? What justifies the claim that Ruth and David's brother belong to the same category? If he is to make such claims, van Manen has an awful lot of explaining to do. But an explanation is not forthcoming.

What is the effect of including such disparate circumstances under the same heading, classifying them as examples of the 'same phenomenon'? Why does van Manen assimilate the experiences of Tommy, Ruth, Martin, Danny, and David's brother into the same category? There are two possibilities. The first is the trivialisation of experiences like Martin's and Ruth's. Because they are the 'same phenomenon' as being dropped off at school, or being left with a babysitter, they can be represented as not deeply significant. This is obviously not van Manen's intention. The second is the very opposite type of assimilation. Since the experiences of Tommy and David's brother are the 'same phenomenon' as being abandoned by a suicidal single parent or a divorced mother, their significance is massively intensified. The underlying message seems to be: dropping off your children at school, or at the day centre, is like abandoning them permanently. It is like committing suicide, absenting yourself for ever after a divorce, or leaving them to the depredations of a cannibalistic witch. It has that kind of significance for the child – and for you as a parent.

This, I suspect, is closer to what van Manen has in mind; and, even before we consider his analysis of the data and his subsequent conclusions about the experience of 'being left or abandoned', it is possible to see a very particular moral view lurking in the shadows. Because phenomenology, let us remember, has moral force. So if leaving your child at a day care centre is like leaving them with a cannibalistic witch, the moral weighting is clearly: 'this is not a good thing to be doing'. I have no doubt van Manen accepts that, in some cases, it is inevitable, and that (as he concedes at one point) school is for the child's own good, not just the parent's convenience. But lumping school, day care, suicide, divorce and cannibals into the same category carries a powerful, emotionally loaded, moral message. It is tantamount to guilt-tripping parents: every time you leave a child with a babysitter, or at the day care centre, you are doing something that is comparable to abandoning them, just as Hansel and Gretel, or Martin Buber, or the daughter in *Sophie's Choice*, were abandoned. Van Manen's own moral understanding of the meaning of 'being left or abandoned' is already implicit in the examples of the 'phenomenon' he has chosen.

A pedagogic understanding

I will, for the moment, skip van Manen's reduction of the 12 descriptions into themes, and home in on his conclusion. The preamble is reasonable, as he observes that 'some children will sometimes have the experience of feeling left, while others may experience the same moment as adventure, as boredom, etc.' (89), a comment that clearly reflects the experience of David, his brother, Julie and Tommy. However, he also toys with the idea that 'perhaps no child ever ought to have the experience of feeling left', even though 'the experience of loneliness is something every child has to face', and 'life is never perfect and we must all battle our personal fears'. But then, abruptly, he focuses on Ruth, the character in Robinson's novel, and finally reveals his own 'pedagogic understanding' of 'being left':

> [Ruth] lives in waiting, in hope. Why? Because the mystery is that in spite of some deep fears, we experience our parents as the solid ground, the home of our existence. A child whose mysterious expectation has been betrayed must learn to deal with a fundamental archetype of human existence: the experience of the vulnerable centre, the broken whole, the neglected hearth, the absent Other. Like Ruth, such a child may for ever be homeless. And we are not even touching upon the overwhelming tragedy of abandoned children living in the major cities of the world. My pedagogic understanding of the theme of 'being left' as 'the experience of homelessness, brokenness' is that insight that permits me to make sense of the text of life.
>
> (90)

This passage is remarkable for a series of shifts, barely noticeable without close attention. We start with Ruth (and let us recall that this is a work of fiction) whose 'mysterious' expectation of her parents as the solid ground has been betrayed. This is generalised to 'a child whose mysterious expectation has been betrayed'; so we are now talking, presumably, of children whose situation is comparable to Ruth's. It is in this context that van Manen refers to the 'broken whole, the neglected hearth, the absent Other'.

The next sentence, 'Like Ruth, such a child...' confirms that the topic is still children-in-a-comparable-situation-to-Ruth. Then, however, we come to an unexpected aside about abandoned children living in the major cities of the world. It is prompted, perhaps, by the mention of homelessness in the previous sentence. There, it is a metaphor for an emotional state. In the aside, by contrast, it appears to be taken literally, and presumably (though van Manen's point is far from clear) refers to children living on the streets. It is not obvious what we are supposed to do with this remark.

Finally, without warning, we arrive at van Manen's pedagogic understanding of the theme of 'being left'. It is unqualified, and no longer refers merely to Ruth, or to children in comparable situations. It is an understanding that applies, on the face of it, to *all* examples of the experience 'being left', because van Manen singles out no exceptions. It is true (and slightly odd) that he now calls it 'being left', whereas he earlier referred to 'the experience of feeling left or abandoned'. However, there is little doubt that this sentence represents his conclusions about the meaning of that phenomenon. It is his understanding of 'being left', not certain *types* of 'being left'; and it informs his ability to make-sense-of-the-text-of-life, not his ability to make-sense-of-*certain-aspects*-of-the-text-of-life. This is a general statement, and there is nothing to suggest that it is not precisely what it appears to be: the main finding of his analysis of the 12 descriptions.[1]

The point is that the language of this 'understanding' is drawn exclusively from his discussion of Ruth and children like her. A child whose 'mysterious expectation' has been betrayed must learn to deal with the experience of the 'broken whole'; and 'such a child may for ever be homeless'. *Such a child.* Not *any* child who has had the experience of 'being left', including those who are dropped off at school or day care. And yet the concepts that apply to 'such a child' are now used (apparently) to characterise *all* children who are in the position of 'being left', even if this is no more than a reference to being left at the day care centre, being left at school, or being left with a babysitter. The slide from (the fictional) Ruth's betrayal by her suicidal single-parent mother to the experience of all (real) children 'being left', if only temporarily, is now complete. They *all* have the experience of 'homelessness, brokenness'.[2]

The theme 'homelessness, brokenness', applied to all children who have the experience of 'being left', carries the same underlying message as the selection of descriptions. If leaving a child in a day care centre and leaving it behind in a concentration camp are the 'same phenomenon'; if dropping a child off at school and abandoning it through suicide are assimilated into the same category; if leaving a child with the babysitter and abandoning it to the depredations of a witch-cannibal count as the same thing ... then the moral weight van Manen attributes to the phenomenon of 'being left or abandoned' is pretty clear. It is the same moral weight as 'homelessness, brokenness'. The implication is that parents should see something deeply wrong about the act of leaving a child with someone else, however temporarily. It is an act that is morally comparable to inflicting homelessness on the child, an act of moral vandalism. Even taking the child to school has a 'brokenness' quality, which parents should obviously be aware of, and reflect upon, every time they do it.

There is (at least to my mind) a strongly evangelical subtext in van Manen's phenomenological example. It is apparent in his selection of descriptions, and it resurfaces in the theme of homelessness-brokenness. However, even if you are inclined to agree with his views, there are two issues that van Manen does not address: first, the fact that a moral position is built into his analysis, even before he gets started; and, second, the fact that his analytical procedures are compromised as a result, because they are a means of vindicating van Manen's own outlook in the guise of data analysis. In this example at least, van Manen is clearly departing from the axiom of resident meaning.

Interpretations and descriptions

Although there is a clear moral position connecting van Manen's selection of cases and his conclusions about the theme of 'being left', there is at least the appearance of an analytical procedure that bridges between the two. This consists of a series of themes, or 'thematic formulations', one for each case. Van Manen introduces this analysis with the following manifesto (86):

> But now we need to see how these examples may open up a deepened and more reflective understanding of the notion of 'feeling left'. In other words, we try to unearth something 'telling', something 'meaningful', something 'thematic' in the various experiential accounts.... What is the essence or *eidos* of the notion of 'being left' and how can I capture this *eidos* by way of thematic reflection on the notion?

One thing worth noticing about this manifesto is that it is couched in language suggestive of something out-there-in-the-world, waiting to be observed, discovered, identified. 'Unearth' implies digging down into the soil for something buried there; 'understanding' implies something that can be misunderstood, something that can be got wrong instead of got right; 'what is the essence ... of the notion of being left' implies that the 'essence' is another sort of object, waiting to be described; the idea that the *eidos* can be 'captured' implies the same thing.[3]

All of which sits uneasily with the claim that 'different readers might discern different fundamental meaning'; that interpretation is 'a free act of seeing meaning'; that a particular interpretation is 'not necessarily more true than another', though it might 'richer or deeper.' The struggle between descriptive phenomenology and interpretive phenomenology continues on every page of the book, even if it is not acknowledged explicitly. The stresses and strains consequent on a view that regards meaning and essence as objects-to-be-described, squeezed into the same frame of reference as a view that regards meaning as an idiosyncratic, personal construct, never completely disappear.

Another thing to notice about the manifesto is the reference to 'experiential accounts'. This is odd for two reasons. First, six of the 12 descriptions are fiction. It is not at all obvious why they count as 'experiential'. They might reflect the meaning of 'being left' to the authors concerned; but fictional works present a particular point of view, and are constructed in order to make that point of view visible to the reader. They have meaning built in, so to speak, so it is not really surprising if an analysis of them 'unearths' that meaning. 'Experiential' they are not.

Second, even the six descriptions that are drawn from real life (apparently: this is not confirmed) include material that cannot be called 'experiential'. Specifically, they include speculation as to the cause of the children's behaviour, speculation that originates either with van Manen himself, or with others. This is odd because, elsewhere in the book, van Manen insists that descriptions should contain neither causal explanations nor any other kinds of interpretation. In the section on protocol writing, for example, he makes suggestions about writing 'lived-experience description': 'You need to describe the experience as you live(d) through it. Avoid as much as possible causal explanations, generalizations, or abstract interpretations' (64). Similarly, in his own case, he notes: 'I try, as Merleau-Ponty says, to give a direct description of my experience as it is, without offering causal explanations or interpretive generalizations of my experience' (54). Yet virtually all of the 12 descriptions in the 'being left or abandoned' example include causal explanations, generalisations, or interpretations.

Consider the description of Patty, who is malleable, obedient, and apparently happy for seven or eight hours in day care, but complaining, hostile and recalcitrant for the first hour or so after she is picked up by her mother or father. The description includes not only the interpretation the two parents place on this behaviour, but van Manen's own speculations. One parent thinks Patty is tired after expending a lot of energy during the day, and is irritable as a consequence. The other thinks she 'needs her mother or father to act out the accumulated frustrations from the day spent in the day-care institution' (81). Van Manen adds his own thoughts:

> Patty's behaviour may have something to do with the daily experience of being left in a place where you cannot be yourself since there is nobody for whom you are really a "self", a unique and very special person.

> (Ibid.)

I don't know what else to call this but speculation about the causes of Patty's behaviour.

Most of the other descriptions include generalisations and interpretations of the same kind, to the extent that it is difficult to understand why van Manen does not comment on the overt inconsistency between his theory and his practice. About Danny, for example, he observes:

> One possible interpretation is that Danny's day-care, in which he spends about ten of his daily waking hours, is not experienced by him as a true home; one cannot feel "left" in a place where one is already left to begin with.

> (82)

Even the fiction is subject to the same treatment. In the case of *Hansel and Gretel*, van Manen cites Bettelheim's interpretation of the fairy tale as symbolising children's need to end their dependency on the parent. However, 'what Bettelheim does not see is that it is not the parent who should abandon the child but the child who should leave the parent' (ibid.). Notice the explicit moral prescription here: the parent *should not* abandon the child. No doubt this is true. But what is astonishing is that van Manen incorporates this view, not merely into his analysis, but into the texts he proposes to analyse.

Interestingly, van Manen suggests that there is something Bettelheim does not 'see', as if the fairy tale contains something that Bettelheim did not notice because he did not observe it closely enough. Does this mean that van Manen's prescriptive account is more accurate than Bettelheim's, because it is based on more careful observation? If so, how does this square with his later claim that one interpretation is no more true than another? Or is it merely 'richer and deeper' than Bettelheim's? In either case, how can we tell? He clearly thinks his interpretation is preferable to Bettelheim's; but he does not explain *why* it is. He does not say whether it is closer to the truth, or whether it is just cuter, sexier, more resonant; and he offers no criteria, no test, that we can apply to determine whether he is correct in this assessment. The conflict between the two distinct approaches to phenomenology – describing objects, or freely inventing meaning – is recognisable on virtually every page of the book.

Thematic formulations

'As I examine the situations,' says van Manen, 'I try some thematic formulations'. What follows this statement is a single sentence, expressing the theme, for each of the 12 descriptions. This is, I take it, the rough equivalent of Giorgi's transformations, in which he distils the meaning of each unit 'more explicitly in language revelatory of the psychological aspect of the lived-through experience'. One main difference is that Giorgi tackles the job piecemeal, transforming each individual 'meaning unit' one at a time. Van Manen, by contrast, dispenses with units, and presents a single 'thematic formulation', which applies to the whole description rather than to any segment of it.

However, despite this difference, there is a marked similarity in their approaches. In neither case is the transition from the story/description to the 'transformed unit'/'thematic formulation' governed by any explicit 'method'. Given the data-description, the transformed meaning (or the thematic formulation) is just what each author says it is, no more and no less. The reader has no means of checking, no means of deciding whether the shift from story to meaning is credible. Giorgi announces, van Manen pronounces … and that's the end of it. Everything is to be taken on trust. Trust me, I'm an expert in phenomenology. Trust me, I'm a scholar. Neither author has a method, though Giorgi claims he has. Van Manen rejects the idea of method, though of course he has a *methodos*. What they have instead is a series of 'meaning' substitutions, entirely dependent on their own say-so.

There is a second very significant difference between Giorgi's example and van Manen's. Giorgi's data consists of stories written by the two workshop participants. Van Manen's data consists of descriptions written by him, sketching out the experience of the children concerned, whether real or fictional. And, as I have already observed, these descriptions are not purely 'experiential', as van Manen implies, but include his own interpretive commentary, incorporated into the data. Consequently, when he begins to 'try some thematic formulations', the job is already done. He did it himself in writing the descriptions.[4]

Recall what he says in Patty's description, for example:

> Patty's behaviour may have something to do with the daily experience of being left in a place where you cannot be yourself since there is nobody for whom you are really a 'self', a unique and very special person.
>
> (81)

Here is his 'thematic formulation' of this case: 'A child who has been left may not experience self in full and unique manner' (86). So van Manen's own interpretation, incorporated into the data-description, now becomes the 'theme'. What a surprise.

Similarly, Danny. Included in the data-description is:

> One possible interpretation is that Danny's day-care, in which he spends about ten of his daily waking hours, is not experienced by him as a true home; one cannot feel 'left' in a place where one is already left to begin with.
>
> (82)

The thematic formulation: 'A child can only feel left from the basis of a relation or situation of at homeness [*sic*] or belonging' (87). So the 'one possible interpretation', is now presented as the theme. According to his manifesto, van Manen has 'unearthed something telling'. He has opened up a 'deepened and more reflective understanding of the notion of "feeling left"'. No, not really. What he has done is simply repeat the interpretation he has already built into the original description.

It's the same with *Hansel and Gretel*. The thematic formulation is: 'A child wants to leave the parents (become independent of the parents) but the child does not want to be left behind by the parents'. This is, actually, an interesting variation because van Manen attributes his own prescriptive interpretation – that it is not the parent who should abandon the child, but the child who should leave the parent – to the child. 'A child wants ... but the child does not want...'. Here, van Manen does not bother to pretend that he has taken a version of the fairy tale and subjected it to an analysis. He has merely compared his own interpretation to Bettelheim's, preferred his own, and then (in the thematic formulation) projected it on to the child, as an expression of what he or she wants.

In some cases, deriving his preferred interpretation from the data requires van Manen to ignore part of the description's content. The 'thematic formulation' for

David reads: 'Being left is the experience of vulnerability, insecurity and incompleteness' (86). However, this presumably can't apply to Tommy, David's brother, who 'hardly takes notice that his parents are leaving' (81). For Tommy, then, being left is the experience of 'hardly noticing'. Similarly, Julie's thematic formulation is: 'Knowing where the parents are provides the child with a sense of control, the security of a home base, being able to reach' (86). But this does not, I take it, apply to Julie's brother, another Tommy, who 'rushes off into the playground' when his father drops him off at school, and apparently has no need to quiz him as to his whereabouts during the day. Although the two brothers do not fit, van Manen has no hesitation in offering a generalisation in each of these cases: 'Being left *is* the experience of...', 'Knowing where the parents are *provides the child* with...'. It is as if he knew what the meaning of 'being left' was going to be before he started – homelessness, brokenness – and cherry-picked the descriptions to make them fit, ignoring anything that didn't. Obviously, I am not claiming that this is what happened. But if I had to provide a 'thematic formulation' of van Manen's procedure, this is the one I would be tempted by. Unlike Giorgi, van Manen seems to have a moral agenda, and he does not shrink from letting it inform his 'hermeneutic phenomenological' reflection.

The daily experience of mothering

Let me now turn to the second example from van Manen's book. It differs from the previous example, because it is based on an account written by somebody other than van Manen himself. The author is referred to as 'Robert's mother', but she is otherwise unidentified. Van Manen introduces her account as a 'lived-experience description ... of the daily experience of mothering' (65). The example is used to illustrate three approaches to 'isolating thematic statements': the 'wholistic or sententious approach', the 'selective or highlighting approach', and the 'detailed or line-by-line approach'. Van Manen's discussion culminates in a 'linguistic transformation' of the description, which is considerably longer than the description itself. The example therefore affords another opportunity to see van Manen's *methodos* in action, starting with the lived-experience account, and moving through the thematic statements to the linguistic transformation.

> Lately I have been wondering if I expect too much of my son. He gets all mixed up in his homework, is overtired, can't think straight, and spends hours doing one straightforward assignment when he should just be relaxing and enjoying family life like all the kids in his class; he has misread the instructions and has to do the whole thing again; he has a thousand ideas for a report on gorillas, but can't seem to get it together to write even the opening sentence. So yesterday I looked at Robbie's cumulative-file at school. I felt guilty in a way, resorting to that, especially since those numbers have so little to say about a person. And my love and hopes for him are unconditional of course; they don't depend on his achievement or IQ scores. But the numbers weren't supposed to tell me whether Rob is

special or not – they were supposed to tell me what to do: whether it is alright for me to tease, prod and cajole him about his homework, and say, 'Hey, you lazy schmuck, get some of this work finished in school instead of fooling around,' or maybe, 'Of course you can't think straight when you're so tired. You'll have to get home earlier and do this homework before supper.'

(95)

The 'wholistic' approach involves writing a single sentence which captures the 'overall meaning' of the text. Van Manen's 'sententious formulation' is: 'A parent needs to be able to know how to act tactfully toward a child in the child's best interest' (94). This does not strike me as an unreasonable summary of the point at issue (although 'to act tactfully' is not an expression I would have chosen myself). The latter part of the text suggests that Robert's mother's main concern is knowing what to do, and deciding whether it would be appropriate to adopt the teasing-prodding strategy that she outlines.

In the 'selective' approach, van Manen picks out certain sentences or phrases 'that seem to be thematic of the experience of parenting', and adds what he takes to be the theme in question. Here are the three sentences/phrases he identifies, together with his thematic comment in each case (94):

'I have been wondering if I expect too much of my son.'
To parent is to distinguish what is good from what is not good for a child

'my love and hopes for him are unconditional of course'
The fundamental experience of parenting is hope.

'they were supposed to tell me what to do'
Parents constantly need to know what to do.

There is no indication of why van Manen thinks that these phrases 'stand out', why he takes them to be especially thematic. And I am not persuaded by his thematic statements. The third one, perhaps, echoes the 'sententious' statement, although the 'constantly' gives it a spin that I do not detect in the original. But I am a bit puzzled by the first and second. The first seems to miss the specific point of the mother's implied question. The second extrapolates wildly from what she actually says, and turns hope into the 'fundamental experience' of parenting. I see no reason for taking this idea as thematic, unless you are already committed to it; and it is difficult to see why hope is any more fundamental than other aspects of being a parent (anxiety, for example).

But it turns out that hope-as-fundamental is the concept van Manen is homing in on. In the 'detailed' approach, he specifies what each sentence of the original account 'shows'. Of the fifth sentence ('And my love and hopes for him are unconditional of course; they don't depend on his achievement or IQ scores'), he says this. '[It] shows that underlying the specific expectations we may cherish, there lies a more fundamental sense of hope' (95). But the fifth sentence quite clearly does not 'show' this. Van Manen's statement misses the point, which is that Robert's mother's love and hope are not conditional on his IQ scores. There may be other reasons for thinking that the sense of hope is fundamental, but the fifth sentence does not provide such a reason. It is non-committal about how fundamental hope is.

When we get to the linguistic transformation, van Manen's apparent insistence on the fundamental nature of hope is suddenly unleashed. Robert's mother's description runs to 18 lines; van Manen's transformation runs to 27, and it is *all* about hope (the word 'hope' and its cognates appears 21 times). Let me give a flavour (96):

> So we must examine how the living with children, at home or at school, is experienced in such a way that we may call it 'hope', 'having hope for children'. The act of hoping, of having hope for a child, is much more a way of being present to the child than a kind of doing. Hope for the parent or the teacher is a mode of being.... But children make it possible for men or women to transcend themselves and to say 'I hope ... I live with hope; I live life in such a modality that I experience children as hope.' This experience of hope distinguishes a pedagogic life from a non-pedagogic one. It also makes clear that we can only hope for children we truly love.... Thus hope gives us pedagogy itself. Or is it pedagogy which grants us hope? Like all great values, their ontological roots seem to merge.

Where on earth did that come from? In Robert's mothers account, hope is mentioned only in passing. She felt guilty about consulting his cumulative-file. Her objective was to find evidence to support (or not) her proposed teasing-prodding strategy. But she recognises that IQ scores say very little about Robert as a person; and she reassures us, parenthetically, that her love and hope are *of course* not conditional on them. That's it. The reference to hope is barely more than a footnote in her account of the problem she faces.

Yet van Manen has transformed this footnote into a paean to hope. It is a mode of being; it makes it possible for women and men to transcend themselves; it distinguishes a pedagogic life from a non-pedagogic one; it gives us pedagogy itself, or pedagogy grants it to us; but, either way, their ontological roots merge. The 'linguistic transformation' is almost completely detached from Robert's mother. It is about 2 per cent her and 98 per cent van Manen, who has evidently abandoned himself to what comes across as a piece of devotional writing, a celebratory flourish, an epistle in the Pauline style on the paramountcy of hope.

So van Manen's personal agenda again swamps his data. He calls this a 'linguistic transformation', but it is more of a substitution, a supersession, a wholesale replacement. Comparing the original text with van Manen's inflated prose, it is impossible to see the transition from description to interpretation as having anything in common with *analysis*. The data is hardly more than a peg on which van Manen can hang a statement of his own values. As with 'being left or abandoned', he clearly has moral priorities of his own.

It is alarming to extrapolate from van Manen to research in nursing, education and psychology. At least with Giorgi there is a sense of method and technique, even if these are illusory. The picture is one of painstaking application, an attempt to distil structures from data. By contrast, consider van Manen. To the extent that his work is used as a model, it legitimates confirmation bias – the search for cases that support one's preconceptions – and a selective approach to the data, ignoring anything that does not fit or that is otherwise uncongenial. Data becomes a Rorschach blot, allowing the projection of personal values on to participants' accounts in the guise of 'thematic statements', 'linguistic transformations', and the '*eidos* of the notion'.

Van Manen's eclectic philosophy can only reinforce this, encouraging the belief that untrammelled, free-range interpretations are phenomenological descriptions of essences, and permitting something invented to be presented as an intrinsic feature of the 'phenomenon'. The point here is independent of whether there are such things as 'essences', or whether the term 'phenomenon' can be rendered unambiguous. It concerns a style of thinking that permits the confusion of 'how it seems to me' with 'how it is', and thereby promotes the substitution of the first for the second. The hermeneutic vision of phenomenology (not just van Manen's) is one of the reasons why this confusion is as extensive as it is.

Meaning still unexplained

Despite his official commitment to the axiom of resident meaning (the meaning of a phenomenon is grasped by coming to grips 'with the structure of meaning of the text', examining every sentence and asking: 'What does this sentence ... reveal about the phenomenon or experience being described?'), van Manen clearly fails to comply with it. Instead, he brings a non-textual resource to the interpretation of the text. In both examples I have considered, this resource consists of his own values.

The contrast with Giorgi is an interesting one. For the most part, Giorgi does try to stick to the text; but the result is that his 'meaning transformations' turn out to be arbitrary synonyms and trivial changes in syntax. Any 'meaning' he produces arises from a vain attempt to compress a story of envy and a story of jealousy into the same 'structure', the same précis. Van Manen, on the other hand, produces 'meaning' in both examples by projecting his own value commitments on to the data. It would appear that, if you stick with the text, you get no meaning, and if you want to derive meaning, you have to go beyond the text.

The obvious question is: how far can this result be extrapolated? Is there some reason why sticking to the text generates no meaning? Or has Giorgi just not done a very good job? Is there some reason why it is necessary to bring an external 'resource' to the process of producing meaning, or is van Manen just in too much of a hurry to vindicate his own moral priorities? Since neither of them provides anything that amounts to a theory of meaning, it is impossible to say.

As far as I'm aware, *no* PQR methodologist has provided a theory of meaning, one that helps us to understand why the axiom of resident meaning is valid (or, alternatively, helps us to understand why it isn't).

So in the next chapter I will suggest one.

Notes

1 Note the bolt-holes van Manen leaves himself. I commented earlier on his writing style, and this is an example. He begins by introducing the experience of 'feeling left or abandoned', but he concludes with 'being left'. He provides no explanation of this change. Perhaps it is insignificant, and he regards the two as identical...? I imagine so, but he does not confirm this. At any rate, the shift makes it possible for him to claim, if he were ever challenged, that 'homelessness, brokenness' does not, after all, represent his overall conclusion about 'the experience of being left or abandoned', since 'being left' is different. Of course, I have no idea whether he would actually say this.

2 Here's another anomaly. On a couple of occasions, van Manen concedes that not all children will have this experience. One of them, as I observed a moment ago, is in the preamble to the analysis. The other occurs in the description of Jeff and his parents: 'To be sure, all children are left sometimes. And children react differently in such situations.' But if children react differently, how can the essence of the experience of 'being left' be homelessness-brokenness? van Manen might have a persuasive answer to this question, but he doesn't tell us what it is.

3 This is the Husserlian part of van Manen's thought. Husserl thought of essences as objects that could be observed, or 'intuited', and described. They are an objective part of the world.

4 Van Manen refers to 'descriptions of several situations which will be treated as concrete occasions for examining the nature and role of meaningful themes in human science' (80). But these situations, as described, are not 'concrete'. The 'meaningful themes' are already built into them.

References

Burhans, L. M., and Alligood, M. R. (2010) 'Quality nursing care in the words of nurses', *Journal of Advanced Nursing*, 66(8), pp. 1689–1697.

Hughes, C., Knibb, W., and Allan, H. (2010) 'Laparoscopic surgery for endometrial cancer: a phenomenological study', *Journal of Advanced Nursing*, 66(11), pp. 2500–2509.

Merleau-Ponty, M. (1962 [1945]) *Phenomenology of Perception*. London: Routledge & Kegan Paul, p. vii, cited in M. van Manen (1990).

Munhall, P. L. (1994) *Revisioning Phenomenology: Nursing and Health Science Research*. New York: National League for Nursing Press.

Sparrow, T. (2014) *The End of Phenomenology: Metaphysics and the New Realism*. Edinburgh: Edinburgh University Press.

van Manen, M. (1990) *Researching Lived Experience: Human Science for an Action Sensitive Pedagogy*. Albany, NY: State University of New York Press.

5 The linguistics of meaning

Both Giorgi and van Manen claim that the aim of PQR is to distil the meaning of a phenomenon from a text; but neither of them explains what kind of thing a 'meaning' is, or how it can be identified. They say only that meaning must be elucidated from the text and nothing but the text. Their examples suggest that, in practice, meaning is whatever Giorgi and van Manen say it is. There are no well-specified and non-arbitrary procedures for achieving the 'transformations in meaning' and 'thematic formulations' that a PQR analysis is said to involve; and at no point does either author provide a theory of meaning, or criteria by which meaning attribution can be tested, checked, or evaluated.

The idiosyncrasies of Giorgi and van Manen's use of 'meaning' are reflected in PQR research reports. No published paper I have seen provides a discussion of the concept, nor is there any indication of how 'meaning' should be operationalised. This is particularly noticeable when 'meaning' is included in the statement of the research aim. Here are some examples from nursing. They are all papers in which the research aim is stated in such a way as to make 'meaning' central.

> ...uncover an understanding of the meaning of quality for practising nurses.

> ...illuminate the meaning of caring in formal care for women with alcohol dependency.

> ...explore the meaning of breast cancer risk for African American women age 40 and under.

> ...investigate the meaning of the experiences of persons with chronic pain.

> ...understand the meaning of being a primary nurse preceptor for newly graduated nurses.

These examples are taken from Burhans and Alligood (2010), Thurang *et al.* (2010), Phillips and Cohen (2011), Hansson *et al.* (2011), and Richards and Bowles (2012) respectively. Given that these statements define the *aim* of the research, one might expect an explanation of what is being sought. Exactly what kind of thing is a 'meaning'? How can it be 'uncovered'? In what way is an 'illumination of meaning' useful? What sort of knowledge does it provide? What will it help you to do more effectively? None of the authors listed above makes much, if any, effort to answer such questions.

So in this chapter I will offer something the PQR writers don't. An analysis of meaning.

In undertaking this analysis, I will draw on corpus linguistics. For many of the book's readers, this will be an unfamiliar technique, so I will begin by providing a brief explanation.[1]

Corpus linguistics

Corpus linguistics is the study of the distribution of words in real-life English. The key idea is that it is possible to determine, empirically, how often certain words occur, and what other words turn up in the same vicinity (known as collocation). A large database, called a corpus, is compiled. The texts that make up the corpus are sampled from academic, newspaper, magazine, fiction, and spoken-language sources, and every word is tagged with a part of speech marker.

Some corpora are specialised. Nottingham University has a corpus that consists of transcripts of patient/professional consultations. Others are more generic. The *British National Corpus* (BNC) is a database of British English texts from the 1980s and 1990s. The *Corpus of Contemporary American English* (COCA) is the US equivalent. It runs from 1990 to 2015, and texts are still being added to it. Both BNC and COCA are both freely available online, hosted at Brigham Young University.

BNC has 100 million words. COCA has 520 million. I said they were large. The new *Google Books: American English 1810–2009* has 155 billion words.

Corpora have several functions. One of them is to identify *collocates* of a selected, or 'target', word – that is, words that appear in the same vicinity as the target. For example, a search for collocates of the word 'big' might specify $(0,1)$, which would (for every instance of 'big' identified in the corpus) pick out the word immediately following it, but ignore all words preceding it. A specification of $(4,2)$ would tabulate all words occurring among the four immediately preceding the target, and all words occurring among the two that immediately follow the target.

Here's a quick and simple example to give an idea of the possibilities. Consider the two adjectives, 'big' and 'large'. They appear more or less synonymous, but are they? And how do we answer this question? Well, one test would be: are they interchangeable? Are they used in the same contexts? Do they qualify the same nouns?

To find out, we turn to the BNC and ask it to identify the nouns which most frequently follow 'big' and 'large'. Table 5.1 shows the top ten $(0,1)$ collocates for each.

By far the most frequent use of 'large' is to qualify abstract nouns of quantity, whereas 'big' qualifies specific and/or relatively concrete items. This is not to say

Table 5.1 BNC (0,1) collocates of 'big' and 'large'

	Big		Large	
1	bang	355	number	1,853
2	man	287	numbers	1,241
3	business	286	part	559
4	house	249	scale	498
5	difference	171	proportion	421
6	ones	148	amounts	377
7	day	146	quantities	352
8	thing	146	extent	342
9	deal	143	amount	337
10	brother	127	areas	323

that it would be wrong to refer to a 'large house' or a 'big number'. It is to say that, in practice, British English markedly prefers 'large number' and 'big house'. This is a question of empirical semantic association, not one of syntactic principle.

Another example. In the last few years I have taken an interest in the literature on spirituality in nursing. One interesting claim often made in this literature is that spirituality and religion are different concepts. Spirituality, it is said, 'includes but is not defined by religion' (Swinton *et al.* 2011). Well, perhaps it is not 'defined' by religion. But does that mean there is no semantic association between the two?

To check, we can look at both COCA and BNC, taking the top ten (4,4) collocates from each. Table 5.2 shows the result.

I have italicised all the religion-related words for both corpora. In COCA, references to religion vastly outnumber non-religious references, and 'religion' is comfortably the top collocate. In BNC, there are considerably fewer instances, but six of the top ten collocates fall into the religious category, and half the instances of 'personal' occur in explicitly religious texts (although 'religion' itself does not appear).

Table 5.2 BNC/COCA (4,4) collocates of 'spirituality'

	COCA		BNC	
1	*religion*	257	personal	10
2	native	129	type	5
3	*Christian*	70	*Christian*	4
4	role	70	*cross*	4
5	*religious*	56	*Benedictine*	3
6	*theology*	51	*mysticism*	3
7	*faith*	49	politics	3
8	science	46	*protestant*	3
9	practice	39	Greek	3
10	Culture	38	*creation*	3

This, I think, tends to undermine the claim that spirituality 'includes but is not defined by' religion. The word 'spirituality' occurs most frequently in discussions of religion, and as a collocate of other religious terms – and this to an overwhelming extent in both countries. You simply cannot use the word without triggering religious associations and connotations. Proposing a redefinition of 'spirituality' that ignores this sociolinguistic fact flies in the face of the empirical evidence. 'Spirituality' is tied to religion in the way that 'best man' is to weddings and 'furlong' is to horse racing.

'Means'

Because the verb and noun forms of the same word often vary in sense (Murphy 2010), I will consider both the noun *meaning* and the verb *to mean*, especially in its third person inflection, *means*. In view of the fact that British and American English do not always coincide semantically, I will refer to both the British National Corpus (BNC) and the Corpus of Contemporary American English (COCA). In this section, I tackle the function of '**means**'. I will deal with '**meaning**' later.

The first thing to do is set aside three irrelevant senses of 'means' and 'mean'. The first is means-as-resources (as in 'means testing' and 'the Ways and Means Committee'). The second is means-as-averages (as in 't-tests compare the means of two different groups'). The third is mean-as-lowly-or-critical-or-stingy (as in 'I think you're very mean'). The first two are *nouns*, the third an *adjective*. All three are clearly unrelated to the *verb* used when we say 'It means the world to me', or 'The word "insouciant" means indifferent, unconcerned, or nonchalant'. In fact, there are four different words here, rather than four senses of the same word.

With the irrelevant senses set aside, we can focus on the verb 'means', the only one of the four that has the noun 'meaning' associated with it.

In both BNC and COCA, the word that most frequently follows 'means' $(0, 1)$ is 'that'. For example, in: 'The train departs at 3:00, which means that we must leave no later than 2:30.' The expression '…means that…' occurs 4,859 times in BNC and 12,570 times in COCA. The next most common collocate is 'to': 'We were discussing what it means to be human'. The expression 'means to' occurs 1,140 times in BNC and 8,953 times in COCA.

Five collocates account for the overwhelming majority of occurrences of 'means' in both corpora:

i   means + 'that'
ii   means + *participle* (keeping, accepting, changing)
iii   means + *comparative quantity adjective* (more, slower, fewer, less)
iv   means + *quantity noun* (something, nothing, a lot, the world)
v   means + to

I will argue that the five constructions fall into two linked but functionally distinguishable groups. The first consists of (i), (ii) and (iii), which are all variations on the same theme. The second consists of (iv) and (v), which are closely related to each other, though not identical. The function of the first group, I will suggest, is to introduce an inference. The function of the second group is to indicate salience. I will analyse the 'inference' group in this section, and deal with the second group later in the chapter.

From here on, I use { } brackets to refer to the various grammatical constructions involving 'means'.

{Means + that} and {means + participle}

First, some examples of these two constructions.

> Belt tightening is the only answer, which **means that** we have to buy less things.
> An hour-a-week meeting **means that** there's not adequate communication.
> Jesus' resurrection **means that** we will not die, not in the eternal sense.
> A fault in the drying cycle **means that** the machine overheats.
> Q1 is defined as a function of Q2, which **means that** Q2 needs to be specified first.
> The complex nature of the reality **means that** a comprehensive analysis is hardly feasible.

> He does understand that a cure **means giving** up drugs.
> Horses need ample fresh water, which **means keeping** water troughs clean and filled.
> But assertiveness also **means accepting** compliments.
> To see things differently **means changing** ourselves in some way.
> Reducing fat in the American diet **means reducing** the amount of animal protein.
> Caring for chronically ill children **means recognising** the family is an interdependent system.

It is apparent that, in some cases, the two constructions are roughly interchangeable. For example, 'Belt tightening means having to buy less things' is the equivalent of 'Belt tightening means that we have to buy less things'; and 'Caring for chronically ill children means that we must recognise the family as an interdependent system' is an alternative to 'Caring for chronically ill children means recognising the family is an interdependent system'. So there is a close relation between the two types of construction.

What is the principle underlying these two 'means' constructions? Consider first {means + participle}. It is fairly clear, even from a cursory inspection, that this construction introduces an inference about the type of action necessary, given a prior condition or requirement. If you want to be cured, you must give up drugs. If you own a horse, you must keep water troughs clean and filled, because horses need lots of fresh water. If you want to learn assertiveness, you must accept compliments. If you wish to see things differently, you must be prepared to change yourself. And so on. {*Means +participle*} specifies (what the speaker/writer believes to be) the action that is necessary if a particular goal is to be achieved. It is the grammatical preface to a practical inference.

Now consider {*means + that*}. As I've already suggested, the belt-tightening example is an alternative to the {*means +participle*} construction; and it, too, clearly introduces a practical inference. The same applies to the 'specifying Q2 first' example: given that Q1 is a function of Q2, it is necessary to specify Q2 first. In both cases, a certain goal (belt-tightening, or defining Q1) requires that a particular action, or series of actions, should be taken: buying less things in one case, specifying Q2 first in the other. So this again illustrates a link between the two constructions.

However, the other four examples are not cases of practical inference. They don't recommend action, or draw attention to the fact that certain actions are necessary in order to achieve a specific goal. But these examples do introduce inferences of a different kind: not practical inference, but inference as to cause and effect.[2] The *consequence* of a fault in the drying cycle is that the machine overheats. A single one-hour meeting per week *leads to* inadequate communication. Jesus' resurrection *brings it about* that we will not die, not in the eternal sense. The complex nature of reality *makes impossible* a comprehensive analysis of it. Each of the verbs in italics is a verb of causation. So the {*means + that*} construction, like the {*means +participle*} construction, introduces an inference. However, it is not necessarily a practical inference. In some cases, it might be; but in a majority of cases, the inference is of the cause-and-effect, one-thing-leads-to-another, type.

There are a few cases in which the {*means + that*} construction introduces an inference that is neither practical nor cause-effect. We might call these logical (including mathematical) inferences. Here are a couple of examples:

$a^2 - b^2 = 5$, which **means** that $(a+b)(a-b) = 5$

The solution isn't 'melba' or 'blame', which **means** that it must be 'amble'

There is no explicitly recommended action here; but neither is there any reference to cause and effect. In both cases, the inference is made on a purely logical basis. In the first example, the inference is based on a procedure for solving quadratic equations; in the second, the writer rules out two anagrams as the solution to a puzzle, and is left with only one remaining possibility.

Finally, there are a few cases in which {*means + that*} takes the form of a clarification of somebody's intentions. For example:

By a smart investment, she **means** that it has saved more money than it cost.
When she says the play was 'interesting', she **means** that it wasn't very good.
Look, when he says he's fine, he **means** that he is positively not fine.

In all these examples, {*means + that*} signals another form of inference – this time, what can be inferred from something someone has said. Here, the inference is not practical, nor logical, nor cause-effect. It is an inference based on an understanding of how another person uses language to convey certain ideas or opinions.

In summary, the {*means + that*} construction is the preface to an *inference*, which may be *cause-effect*, *practical*, *logical*, or *clarifying*. In the case of the practical type, {*means + that*} can be replaced by a grammatical alternative, {*means + participle*}, which introduces the same kind of inference, using the participle to specify the kind of action necessary or recommended.

For all types of {*means*} inference, there is a relevant theory – in some cases, we might want to call it 'knowledge' – that underpins the inference itself. Call this, a convenient shorthand, the *background theory*. In the case of a *cause-effect* inference, the theory in question will be about the mechanisms at work, or at least confirmable generalisations implying those mechanisms. 'A fault in the drying cycle means that the machine overheats' presupposes a background theory concerned with the working of the machine. Similarly, 'Jesus' resurrection means that we will not die, not in the eternal sense' implies a theological theory of cause-and-effect, according to which there are various procedures adopted by God, such that the resurrection of Jesus brings about eternal life for the 'we' referred to.

With the *logical* type of inference, the relevant theory might be mathematics – in the example above, it is algebra – or some other system in which a deductive inference can be made. In the second example, there are three possible anagrams, in English, of the letters [m b l e a]; and if, in a crossword puzzle, two of them can be ruled out, that leaves only the third.

The *clarifying* type depends on a theory about a particular person's mode of communication, and her use of language especially. This theory will, in turn, be supported by relevant evidence, and mainly by a familiarity with how she has behaved in comparable situations in the past. For example, 'When she says the play was "interesting", she means that it wasn't very good' is based on an understanding of the individual being referred to: her use of irony, her preference for euphemism, her unwillingness to hurt someone else's feelings, or whatever.

Finally, *practical* inference is almost always based on a cause-effect theory, or occasionally (as with the Q2 example) a logical theory. The water troughs must be kept clean and filled because horses need lots of fresh water (and if they don't get it, they will become dehydrated, or even sick). Animal proteins are causally responsible for the fat in American diets, so reducing animal proteins is necessary if the diet is to be improved. Drugs compromise a person's health, so if the patient wants to be cured (of the relevant illness), she will have to give them up. And so on. These are all cases of practical reasoning. Assuming you do not want your horse to fall sick, assuming you want to be cured, then the physiological facts demand that you keep the water trough clean and filled, and give up the drug habit. A certain aspiration, combined with a certain theory about how things work, leads to an inference about what you must do. Putting it in formulaic terms: goal + causal theory = an inference about necessary action.

The theory supporting the inference is held, rather obviously, by the speaker, who may assume that others hold it as well. In some cases, as with the horses-needing-water example, this assumption is very likely to be true. But not necessarily. For example, not everybody will share the theological theory according to which the resurrection of Jesus ensures that 'we will not die in the eternal sense'. So the 'means that', in this case, refers to a theory espoused by the speaker (and no doubt others) but not by everyone. We might say, then, that the 'meaning' that the resurrection of Jesus has for the speaker is not a 'meaning' that it will have for all those who read the sentence. Another example. If someone said 'Giving your child the MMR vaccination means that you increase the risk of autism' (some people still do say this), I would argue that the evidence shows, conclusively, that they are wrong.

Here is one corollary of this line of thought. I have argued that the kind of meaning represented by the {*means + that*} and {*means + participle*} constructions refers to an inference that is based on a theory held, implicitly or explicitly, by the speaker. The inference may be what I have termed practical, causal, logical or clarifying; but the background theory will almost always be of the cause-effect, one-thing-leading-to-another type. In the context of these two constructions, then, anyone who presumes to tell us what something means is drawing on a causal theory that she believes, but that some members of her audience might not share. If they don't share it, both the theory and the inference it supports will be subject to challenge.

What this corollary rules out is an account of meaning that implies that it is independent of a specific theory; that it is the kind of thing a 'meaning expert' can tell us about; that it is something which can be distilled through 'meaning transformations'; that it is something a phenomenologist (such as Giorgi) or a scholar (such as van Manen) can be trusted to elucidate; that it is a quality belonging to the world that can be seen, intuited, recognised or discerned by the properly trained. In other words, what it appears to rule out is the axiom of resident meaning.

If this is correct, it makes sense of the examples that both Giorgi and van Manen present, which I discussed in Chapters 3 and 4. It explains why there is no 'method', or even a *methodos*, which can be used to identify and 'transform' meaning, or to write 'exhaustive' statements on the 'essential meaning' of the 'phenomenon'. It explains why neither author can provide even a cursory sketch of the method he claims to adopt. It explains why van Manen appears to project his own views into the analysis, and into his selection of data, and why Giorgi makes a farrago of jealousy and envy. There is just nowhere else for meaning to come from: a background theory that supports the inference *X means that Y*. On the analysis I have just outlined, there is no such thing as *the* meaning of anything. There are only inferences about X, based on various background theories that the speaker entertains.

Of course, this corollary applies just to meaning as represented by the constructions {*means + that*} and {*means + participle*}. It is possible that {*meaning + of*} is different. So a discussion of that construction is necessary as well. More of that in a while.

The *{means + comparative quantity adjective}* construction

We can now take a brief look at comparative adjectives of quantity. Some examples from COCA:

> Tourism is still down; that **means fewer** jobs and lower wages
> Being a breastfeeding mother also **means less** ovarian cancer and fewer hip fractures
> Scarce ice **means fewer** perches from which polar bears can search for seals
> It's a concentrate, which **means less** weight to bring aboard and store

Even at a glance, it is possible to see that *{means + comparative quantity adjective}* introduces another inference. All four examples spell out the consequence of something. The consequence of tourism being down is that there will be fewer jobs and lower wages; the consequence of scarce ice is that polar bears have fewer hunting perches. As with *{means + participle}*, this construction can readily be translated into *{means + that}*: 'It's a concentrate, which means that there is less weight to bring aboard'. To that extent, then, the construction is effectively a variant of *{means + that}*. The nature of the inference is something-that-follows-from-something-else. In the first two examples, this is a cause-effect relation. In the third and fourth, it is not a question of one thing causing another; but an implication of the situation described is none the less indicated. The scarcity of ice does not, strictly speaking, *cause* fewer perches; but fewer perches are a *consequence* of scarce ice, and one which someone reading about the effects of climate change on polar ice might not necessarily, or not immediately, recognise.

In this construction, then, as in the others I have already discussed, 'means' introduces an inference. It is, in effect, a grammatical alternative to *therefore* or *consequently*. One might say: 'Tourism is still down; therefore, there will be fewer jobs'. Or one might say: 'Tourism is still down; that means fewer jobs'. Similarly, one might say: 'We have a meeting for an hour per week; consequently, there will be inadequate communication'. Or one might say: 'A meeting for an hour a week means that there will be inadequate communication'. And 'Jesus was resurrected; therefore, we will not die in the eternal sense' is a functional substitute for 'Jesus' resurrection means that we will not die in the eternal sense'.

In all these constructions, 'means' does no more than introduce an inference. It is, as I shall say, an *inference marker*.

Philosophical interlude

This concludes the analysis of the verbal constructions, *{means + that}*, *{means + participle}* and *{means + comparative quantity adjective}*, whose function is that of an inference marker. The analytical work that still needs to be done is to consider the *{means}* constructions that indicate salience. I also want to discuss the noun *meaning*, and the constructions that take the form *{meaning + of}*.

However, before proceeding, I would like to pause and take stock. The main conclusion so far is that a primary function of the verb 'mean' is to signal an inference – frequently, though not always, a causal one. The inference-marker analysis, I want to suggest, applies equally to the constructions that take the form {*meaning* + *of*}. Later, I will show how this works; first, however, I want to explain the basic idea that is emerging, and comment briefly on its ramifications.

In the rest of this section, then, I invite the reader to suspend disbelief temporarily, and imagine that the inference-marker analysis can be applied to the 'meaning of...' constructions as well as to 'means...'. In fact, assume that it applies more or less across the board – that it is true of all, or most, relevant senses of the words 'means' and 'meaning'.[3]

The meaning-as-inference analysis is at odds with a familiar picture of meaning. This picture – or rather a series of related pictures – is derived from some classic theories of word meaning, particularly those associated with the logician/philosopher, Gottlob Frege.[4] In earlier theories, the meaning of a word was identified with the object it refers to, or the class of objects it refers to. The meaning of 'chair', on this account, is either a specific chair, or the set of things to which the word is correctly applied – in other words, chairs. This theory doesn't work, because some words refer to things that don't exist: 'unicorn', 'phlogiston', 'elf', and so on. Because there are no such things as unicorns, the meaning of 'unicorn' cannot be an object or a set of objects.

In Frege's account, there is, in addition to a *word* and an *object*, a third entity: *sense* (which is the usual translation of Frege's *Sinn*). On this view, the meaning of a word is its sense, not the object; and the sense permits the word to *refer* to the objects (if any) that it is used to describe. Sense is pictured as a sort of intermediate layer between the object and the word. The sense is 'attached' to the word, and the word may (or may not) refer to an object or set of objects. 'Chair' and 'unicorn' both have a sense, but only 'chair' *refers*. It can be used to label things that actually exist.

The picture of meanings as entities, occupying the space between words and objects, is encouraged by the way Frege talks about 'a realm of sense', 'a realm of reference', and a 'realm of word and sentence'. This way of speaking inevitably conjures up an image of related dimensions, somehow attached to each other; and it appears to grant an ontological status to 'meaning' that is roughly the equivalent of the ontological status possessed by words and objects, both of which are literally things: either marks on the page, or the various things, events and processes that can be referred to.

At the same time, however, the sense is something very like an attribute of the word. The word's sense 'belongs' to the word, almost part of it; it is somehow 'glued' to the word (Wilson 2006). On this view, then, a 'sense' is simultaneously an *entity* – one of countless similar entities in a 'realm of sense' – and an *attribute*, a property the word has. Quite how it can be both at once is one of the problems associated with this picture of language.[5]

The trouble is: once this image is adopted, it becomes difficult to think about meaning any other way. Although the idea of a 'realm' of meaning is intrinsically peculiar – Where is it? What kind of things are meanings? Exactly how are they attached to words? – the temptation to think in terms of quasi-objects, somehow glued to words, is very strong. In this way, 'meaning' becomes rather mysterious. As Dummett (1973: 154) suggests: 'the realm of sense is a very special region of reality; its denizens are, so to speak, things of a very special sort'. Words clearly have meanings; but it is just not clear what we are saying when we make this claim. Words have … what? And what kind of 'having' is that?

The technical and philosophical problems associated with Frege's theory are of no particular concern to us here. But the picture of meaning as a special 'realm' is a hypnotic one. Frege applies the concepts of sense and reference to words or, more generally, signs. But suppose we get the idea that 'meaning' is an attribute not just of words, but of 'phenomena' and experiences. Suppose we think that a 'phenomenon' has a 'meaning' in the same way that a word does. Obviously, this meaning is not something that can be looked up in a dictionary; but, if the 'realm of meaning' is preserved as an analogy, then we are likely to believe that a phenomenon's meaning is something that can be identified and described, just as a word's meaning can, and that it is somehow 'attached' to the phenomenon in the way that a word's meaning is 'attached' to the word. Like word meaning, a phenomenon's meaning is both an entity and an attribute.

Personally, I don't think this picture makes a lot of sense. It is impressionistic at best, and I cannot see how to answer the hard questions: What, precisely, is the kind of meaning that is typically attached to a phenomenon, and what form does this 'attachment' take? However, these are not the questions I want to dwell on here. Instead, let me emphasise that the analysis presented so far in this chapter is completely at odds with the picture of meaning I have just sketched. Meanings, on this account, are not a 'realm' of entities attached to phenomena, in the way that word-meanings are attached to words. Rather, 'meaning' language is used to introduce inferences based on theories.

Consider the earlier example: 'assertiveness means accepting compliments'. In the corpus linguistics analysis, the 'meaning' of assertiveness is not conceived as a mysterious something that is attached to the 'phenomenon', and that can be made known by a scholar or 'meaning expert'. It is not conceived as any kind of entity. According to the inference-marker analysis, to say that 'assertiveness means accepting compliments' is to make an inference about the *implications* of being assertive. Similarly, to say that 'an hour-a-week meeting means that there will not be adequate communication' is to make an inference about the *effect* that meetings lasting only one hour a week will have. And to assert that the meaning of the Resurrection is that we will not die in the eternal sense is to make an inference, based on a theological theory, about the Resurrection's *outcome*.

In short, instead of an ontologically dubious 'realm of meaning' attached to 'phenomena', the analysis presented here shows that talk about 'meaning' is a way of introducing inferences based on theories. To oversimplify a bit, 'means that' is the functional equivalent of 'therefore'. And this analysis (as I will suggest later) applies to almost every use of 'means' and 'meaning'. The analysis replaces a mysterious 'realm of sense' with a simple linguistic function: the words, 'means' and 'meaning' do the same job as 'therefore'.

Figure 5.1 (which I'll repeat in extended form later) makes the same point. It might not make complete sense yet, because I have still to undertake an analysis of the {*meaning + of*} constructions. However, it will help to emphasise the point that virtually all uses of 'means' and 'meaning' can be translated, more or less, into 'therefore'.

The figure does not include the {*means + to*} construction or the {*means + quantity noun*} construction, both of which indicate degree of salience. I will discuss these constructions later, following the analysis of the {*meaning + of*} constructions. My intention at this juncture is only to summarise the inference-introducing function of 'means' and 'meaning'.

In the next section, then, I will look at the {*meaning + of*} constructions. These fall into two categories: {*meaning + of + general concept*} and {*meaning + of + particular*}.

'Meaning'

The top 50 collocates (0,3) of {*meaning + of*} fall into four main categories: linguistic items; abstract nouns with a political, religious and existential flavour; laws and statutes; symbolic items. Examples:

Linguistic	'word', 'expression', 'term', 'sentence', 'phrase', 'utterance', 'verb', 'language'
Abstract	'life', 'truth', 'existence', 'democracy', 'freedom', 'marriage', 'religion', 'justice'
Statutory	'section', 'article', 'act', 'statutory', 'section 21'
Symbolic	'parable', 'poem', 'symbol', 'dream'

There is an interesting difference between the BNC and COCA. While linguistic items form the largest group in both of them, statutory references play a much more significant role in the BNC, while abstract nouns play a much more significant role in COCA. In BNC, 'life' is the only abstract noun to appear in the top 30 collocates. In COCA, the top 30 include 'life' (the most common of all), 'democracy', 'existence', 'marriage', 'citizenship', 'justice', 'success', 'freedom', 'religious', 'religion', 'revelation', 'constitution'. {*meaning + of*} in BNC, then, has to do largely with linguistic and legal items; whereas in COCA, it has to do with linguistic items, together with cultural, political and religious concepts.

Just to emphasise this point, consider the top ten collocates (0,1) of {*meaning + of*} – that is, the list of words which most frequently follow 'meaning of'. In BNC, this list is:

section, terms, life, article, words, pain-language, history, bye-law, ethical, meaning.

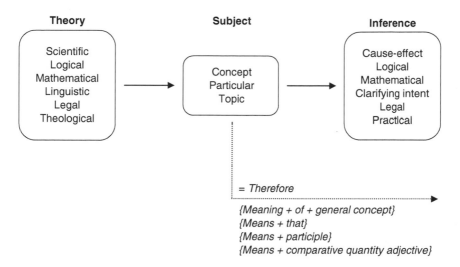

Theory	Subject	Inference
Scientific Logical Mathematical Linguistic Legal Theological	Concept Particular Topic	Cause-effect Logical Mathematical Clarifying intent Legal Practical

= *Therefore*

{Meaning + of + general concept}
{Means + that}
{Means + participle}
{Means + comparative quantity adjective}

Figure 5.1 'Means' and 'meaning': interim model.

This list includes five linguistic items, three statutory items, and two broadly cultural items ('history', and 'ethical'). Contrast this with the COCA list:

> life, Christmas, words, human, democracy, success, freedom, marriage, citizenship, section.

The mix is very different: one linguistic item, one statutory item, seven cultural items, and the hard-to-classify 'success'. The BNC collocates are largely about language and legal frameworks. In COCA, overwhelmingly, they are about political and cultural issues. Any discussion of 'meaning', in whatever context, must surely take account of the discrepancy between British and American uses.

Putting this question aside, however, we can consider some of the contexts in which {*meaning + of*} appears in one of the corpora. As an example, I will consider 'marriage', appearing eighth in the list of words that most frequently follow {*meaning + of*} in COCA; and 'Christmas', which appears second.

> A man-woman meaning is a widely shared public **meaning of** marriage
> to create a gay marriage is to change the **meaning of** marriage
> all the heterosexuals in this state have been deprived of the basic **meaning of** marriage
> communities of faith debate the theological **meaning of** marriage and a viable sexual ethic
> an opportunity to be reminded of the **meaning of** marriage in the Catholic sense
> religious teaching endorses a **meaning of** marriage centred on having and rearing children

the unitive **meaning of** marriage cannot be separated from the procreative

cut marriage off from its religious and natural roots, and the true **meaning of** marriage is lost

personal freedom and the acceptability of divorce have changed the very **meaning of** marriage

Americans are battling about who owns the **meaning of** marriage

the **meaning of** Christmas for me – a bringing together of faith and love

He sent Jesus to change and comfort hearts, and that is the **meaning of** Christmas

the Incarnation, the immigration of God, teaches us the redemptive **meaning of** Christmas

displaying menorahs but not Nativity scenes is diluting the **meaning of** Christmas

the real **meaning of** Christmas is not the birth of Jesus, it's his death

the **meaning of** Christmas: our gifts celebrate the birthday of an infant, the Christ

they've lost the true **meaning of** Christmas, because it's about giving presents

She knew that the real **meaning of** Christmas was love

learns the true **meaning of** Christmas after being visited by three ghosts

Scholars studying the cultural **meaning of** Christmas have interpreted the festival as an interlude

One interesting difference between these two examples is that 'marriage' is a general concept with numerous instances, while 'Christmas' refers to one specific thing, a particular religious festival. Other examples (all listed in COCA) of general concepts might include: success, caring, sacrifice, friendship, liberal, democracy, citizenship, religion. Other examples of named particulars would be: Christianity, Jesus, Genesis, Easter, Thanksgiving, life, existence, and 9/11. It turns out that {*meaning + of*} works in a subtly different way in the two types of construction.

The {*meaning + of + general concept*} construction

I will start with the {*meaning of*} a general concept, in this case marriage. The COCA sample is clearly influenced by the debate, in recent years, about same-sex marriage; but that does not prevent us from seeing what sort of claims are being made here. In six of the ten examples, criteria are being identified, whether implicitly or explicitly, for determining what counts as a marriage. In the first two, it is claimed that a necessary condition for counting something as a marriage is that it should involve a woman and a man, not two people of the same sex. The same criterion is implied by the third example, although the thought is expressed in rather melodramatic language. Similarly, the fifth and sixth examples specify another criterion: that, for something to count as a marriage, it should involve procreation and children. The seventh, in referring to the 'Catholic sense', hints at the same criterion. Of course, the 'procreation' criterion entails the 'man/woman' criterion, although this is not made explicit.

The remaining examples illustrate a difference between {*means + that*} and {*means + participle*} on the one hand, and {*meaning + of + general concept*} on the other. In the first two constructions, the speaker endorses the inference and the background theory on which it is based. By contrast, in {*meaning + of + general concept*}, this kind of speaker endorsement is not necessarily required. The fourth example does not commit itself to any particular criterion, but merely refers to communities of faith discussing the options. Equally, the tenth refers to comparable debates as a battle, but again does not commit the writer to any particular position. This is a distinction connected to the grammar. {*Means + that*} introduces an inference that is endorsed by the writer. However, {*meaning + of + general concept*} makes it possible to refer to various claims that are made, but without specifying what they are, and without subscribing to any of them. 'Communities of faith debate the theological meaning of marriage' implies that there are several views being debated, but does not explain what they are, and does not appear to take sides.

It is clearly very useful to have a way of referring to claims without being committed to endorsing them. Apart from anything else, it makes it possible to make sociological and anthropological observations, such as 'Americans are battling about who owns the meaning of marriage', and 'Scholars are studying the cultural meaning of Christmas'. But this possibility – mentioning the debate, without engaging in it – should not distract attention from the principal use of {*meaning + of + general concept*}, which is to specify a criterion for what *counts*, or should count, as an instance of the general concept.

As I have suggested, {*means + that*} and {*means + participle*} presuppose a background theory that supports the inference introduced by the construction. Similarly, where a claim about identifying criteria is endorsed, there will be a background theory associated with {*meaning + of + general concept*} that explains or justifies the claim in question. For example, the view that a necessary condition of marriage is 'having and rearing children' is justified by 'religious teaching'. It is not clear what the background justification for the 'union of a man and a woman' view is; but it might be religious teaching again (as this type of union is ordained by God). Alternatively, it might be lexicographical: 'to create a gay marriage is to change the meaning of marriage' could just be a reference to a shift in semantics. A third possibility is that the justification might be social. 'A man-woman meaning is a widely shared public meaning of marriage' could be invoking a culturally entrenched usage as justification for specifying the man-woman union as a criterion. In all three cases, the male-female criterion appears to be endorsed, but for reasons that vary: religious teaching, what the dictionary says, or a shared social expectation.

Other background theories include: the idea that a union of a man and a woman is an 'intrinsic good'; the claim that nothing is more important to the public weal than 'maintaining a set of social conditions in which children being raised by their moms and dads is the norm'; the view that personal fulfilment requires participation in a 'biological, one-flesh unity'; and so on (George and Elshtain 2006).

As with {*meaning + that*} or {*meaning + participle*}, the background theory might be shared with the audience, or then again it might not. Rhetorically, however, the writer implies that it is, in fact, shared. The use of the definite article 'the' – and qualifiers such as, the 'true' meaning', the 'basic' meaning, and the 'core' meaning – create the impression of something incontrovertible. This is a grammatical illusion. The background theory is always subject to challenge by those who disagree with it. So, despite phrases such as 'the true meaning of marriage', there is no such thing as *the* meaning.

If there is an implied background theory providing a justification for the criterion proposed, there is also an implied inference. Unlike {*means + that*}, where the inference is explicit, and where the construction itself introduces that inference, in {*meaning + of + general concept*} the inference is implicit (although it is usually spelled out elsewhere in the same text). Here, the implied inference is that there should not be legal provision for same-sex marriages, or that same-sex marriage is always morally wrong.

Let me briefly illustrate these observations by referring to some other examples.

> The **meaning of** organisation is to create structures that fuel radically meaningful work, life, and play

Here, then, is a proposed criterion for what counts as an organisation. An inspection of the relevant text reveals the background theory: building these structures will ensure that production, consumption and exchange will achieve greater peaks of prosperity.

> The **meaning of** respect is to treat everyone with the same degree of respect, regardless of rank or status

The proposed criterion is an equality of respect, rather than something that is targeted at specific people or groups. The background theory suggests that this will make one a better leader.

> The **meaning of** revolution is not just political upheaval but an attack on the economic system

A necessary criterion of revolution is attempting to destroy the economy. The background theory is that this is the strategy of the totalitarian left. If, in the first two examples, the implied practical inference is to create the relevant structures (even if that is a rather hazy project), and to respect everyone equally, the implication here is to be vigilant, and to snuff out the totalitarian left's activities whenever they are detected.

In summary, then, the {*meaning* + *of* + *general concept*} construction typically specifies a criterion, or necessary condition, for something to count as an instance of the concept; implies a background theory that justifies the criterion proposed; and further implies a practical inference concerning what should or should not be done. A derivative use of the same construction makes it possible to refer to debates about the merits of different criteria, but without endorsing any particular point of view.

It is worth noting that there is, in this respect, both a symmetry and an asymmetry between {*meaning* + *of* + *general concept*} and {*meaning* + *that*} or {*meaning* + *participle*}. In both cases, there is a theory hovering in the background that justifies an inference, which may or may not be shared with the audience. But there are two differences. One is that {*meaning* + *of* + *general concept*} leaves both the background theory and the inference implicit, while {*meaning* + *that*} not only makes the inference explicit, but is designed to introduce it. The other is that {*meaning* + *of* + *general concept*} explicitly proposes a criterion, while {*meaning* + *that*} and {*meaning* + *participle*} connect the background theory and the inference directly, in the context of a hypothetical imperative.

The {*meaning* + *of* + *particular*} construction

I can now turn to the second set of examples, illustrating the {*meaning* + *of* + *particular*} construction. It would be convenient if the analysis of {*meaning* + *of* + *general concept*} could be applied equally to this construction; but there is an obvious problem that blocks this. Proposing a criterion for something to count as a member of a particular category – marriage, revolution, respect – doesn't make sense when we are talking about the meaning of an individual item, something of which there is only one, and which has a name. Christmas is not a class; neither are Napoleon or the Crimean War.

However, it is not hard to spot what {*meaning* + *of* + *particular*} achieves. There may not be a criterion for membership, but there is still a background theory; and with this construction it is rather more in the foreground. In effect, the {*meaning* + *of* + *particular*} construction points towards a theory of why there is such a particular in the first place. In the case of Christmas, the background theory tells us why there is such a festival. It tells us what its function is, where it came from, why it's there.

The examples listed earlier do not agree about this. They exhibit different theories. For example, one of them suggests that Christmas exists because of the Incarnation, while another implies that it is the birth of Christ, the Nativity, with which it is associated. A third affirms that Christmas has something to do, not with the birth of Jesus, but with his death – since death is only made possible by birth. Christmas is celebrated, then, because the Nativity is the beginning of a death, not because the birth is of intrinsic interest in itself. In one example, the fact that presents are exchanged suggests that we have forgotten the real reason why this date is celebrated. In another, the exchange of gifts is part of the celebration. In yet another example, neither the birth, nor the death, nor the present giving is mentioned. Instead, the background theory is God's intention in 'sending' Jesus: to change and comfort hearts. On that view, Christmas is celebrated to keep alive a certain message, not for subtle reasons centred on Jesus' birth, death or resurrection.

The fact that there are different theories explaining why Christmas is celebrated is, of course, consistent with the hypothesis that there is no such thing as *the* 'meaning of' something. As before, the grammar is misleading, with the definite article being boosted by 'real' or 'true' in order to convey that there is only one *accurate* theory, and that the speaker/writer is presenting it. All other theories can be discounted. So the rhetoric of such claims exploits the syntactic illusion of singularity. We don't need meaning experts to decode 'the meaning'. We just need to recognise that people have different theories, different beliefs.

In the examples mentioned so far, the explanatory theory has been explicit, and the practical inference implicit. However, there are a couple of examples in which the practical inference is signalled more clearly: love in one case, and the bringing together of faith and love in the other.

I should also note, in passing, that {*meaning + of + particular*} has a non-committal version, just as the {*meaning + of + general concept*} construction does, and for the same reasons. It is clearly useful to be able to refer to various theories, and the fact that they are held, without committing the speaker to any one of them. There are no clear instances of this in the listed examples, but it is possible to find them in COCA: 'a play about the meaning of Christmas'; 'on an adventure to discover the meaning of Christmas'; 'our eighth grade teacher assigned a composition on the meaning of Christmas'. However, it is interesting that these examples are relatively rare: of 70 instances in COCA, 43 include the booster adjectives 'true' or 'real', and most of the rest have some particular theory clearly in mind.

As with {*meaning + of + general concept*}, I will refer briefly to a few other examples.

> The working class will recognise itself as the **meaning of** history.
> The **meaning of** the cross: God so loved the world that He gave his only begotten son.
> The **meaning of** 9/11? To create and sustain an obsessive hatred of Muslims.
> The **meaning of** life is not to rule but to render service to one's neighbour.

The background theory in the first two should be fairly clear: one Marxist, the other theological. In the third, a political theory is implied, explaining why 9/11 has become a unique symbol (rather than just a shorthand for a series of events). In the fourth – one of the very few instances in which a meaning of life is specified, not just referred to in a non-committal way – it is the implied inference that is explicit, not the background theory. Even so, the language in which the inference is couched ('neighbour') suggests a probable source for the corresponding theory.

To summarise: the {*meaning* + *of* + *particular*} construction alludes, implicitly or explicitly, to a theory that accounts for the existence of the individual item in question. The theory may be causal, or it may specify a function, or it may be a story about origins; but in all cases it is implied that this is the truth of the matter, even though there will typically be several non-identical explanations of the same thing. In this construction, it is normally the theory that is most evident, while inferences are commonly – but not invariably – left implicit. As before, there is a non-committal version that permits reference to one or more theories without necessarily committing the speaker/writer to a specific position.

If the other 'means' and 'meaning' constructions considered up to now are the functional equivalent of 'therefore', the {*meaning* + *of* + *particular*} construction is the functional equivalent of 'because'.

Salience

The analysis so far has focused on the inference-marker function of 'means' and 'meaning', a function exhibited by some of the {*means*} constructions and by the {*meaning* + *of*} construction. However, I have not yet looked at two other constructions that were identified earlier: {*means* + *quantity noun*} and {*means* + *to*}. In this section, I will tackle both of these, suggesting that they indicate salience.

The {means + quantity noun} construction

This construction appears in one kind of PQR question, 'What does… X mean to you?', and in popular culture: 'Winning this award means everything to me.' Here are some examples from COCA:

> My faith **means a lot** to me.
> Each time I perform it, it **means something** special.
> Killing **means nothing** to him.
> It **means the world** to me to have won the Orange Bowl.

In these examples, a statement is made about how important something is to the person concerned, how far she cares about it, whether it matters. 'It means nothing to me' indicates that I am indifferent, that it has no importance, and does not affect me emotionally. 'It means something to me' indicates that I do regard it as important. 'It means a lot to me' attaches a greater degree of importance to it; and 'It means the world to me' attaches more importance again. But these are very vague claims. They are not precise measures of how much something matters; and, partly for this reason, they can often be insincere. When a wealthy sportsperson who has won many competitions says, of a minor television award, 'This means a lot to me', we can be forgiven for wondering whether she is genuinely stirred.

I think this construction is a bit tangential, compared to the inference-introducing constructions; but it should not be dismissed. When the researcher begins an interview by asking, for example, 'What does quality nursing care mean to you?' (Burhans and Alligood 2010), it is not obvious that the respondent will *not* hear this as 'How important is quality nursing care to you?', and that what she says will not to some degree reflect this interpretation. So the 'how important' sense of 'means' is at least hovering in the air when this sort of question is asked. I will return to it briefly at the end of the chapter.

The {means + to} constructions

When this combination turns up in the corpora, 'means' is often being used in the 'resource' sense. The combination is typically followed by a verb such as 'achieve' or 'deliver: 'the political means to achieve a united Ireland'; 'an effective means to deliver services to all students'. As before, I shall set aside this 'resource' noun as irrelevant to the 'means/meaning' sense we are exploring.

In COCA, by far the most frequent $(0, 1)$ collocate of {means + to} is 'be'; and the same word is also common in BNC, though not quite to the same extent. In both corpora, there is also a significant, but far less frequent, combination: {means + to + pronoun}, as in: 'You have no idea what this means to me'. In this section, then, I will discuss both constructions: {means + to + pronoun} and {means + to + be}.

Many examples of {means + to + pronoun} function as a rough alternative to {means + quantity noun}.

> You just don't know what this **means to me**.
> I want to let him know how much he **means to me**.
> You know what music **means to me**.
> I'll show you exactly how little that **means to me**

These are roughly synonymous with expressions such as 'This means a lot to me' and 'This means so much to me'. The frequent use of 'know', whether in the positive or negative, appears to be a method of emphasising the degree of salience. 'You just don't know what this means to me' clearly implies: 'It means a great deal; more than you realise'.

There are some uses of {means + to + pronoun} that have a different function. These examples are from COCA:

> Professional **means to me** not making mistakes.
> What Elvis **means to me** is memories, sweet memories.
> What political correctness **means to me** is related to justice.
> Friendship and the will to live … that's what skiing **means to me**.

In these instances, the speaker specifies something that she *associates* with the concept, activity or person in question. These associations are clearly personal, although they might be shared with other people. Many music lovers have good memories of Elvis Presley; however, others may be indifferent or antipathetic. Political correctness may be linked to the idea of justice for some people, but for others it is associated with intolerance, repressive liberalism or cultural Marxism. So 'What X means to me' refers, in its associative function, to something the speaker connects with X, something that X puts her in mind of, something that she regards as a consequence or a cause of X.

I will say more about association when I turn to {*means + to + be*} in a moment. But I think it is clear that there is an overlap between the associative function and the inference-introducing function. Where the association refers to something that, according to the speaker, is a consequence of X, or a practical requirement of X, or a cause of X, this overlap is particularly obvious. For example:

> They booed him all through the ceremony. That **means to me** that there's a level of incivility.
> The machine overheated. What that **means to me** is a fault in the wiring.
> I failed the test. What that **means to me** is I'll be ridiculed.
> What Veterans Day **means to me** is to honour those young people.

All these examples involve an inference; but, equally, they could all be described as associative: what the speaker associates with booing, overheating, failing, or Veterans Day. The first and second are causal inferences: incivility caused the booing; faulty wiring caused overheating. The third is an inference about an effect: the effect of failing will be ridicule. The fourth is a practical inference: on Veterans Day one should honour those young people.

An overlap between the inference-marking function and the associative function is also characteristic of the {*means + to + be*} construction, which I will now consider before I attempt to summarise the whole discussion.

The {*means + to + be*} construction

In both COCA and BNC, the word that most frequently follows this combination is 'human' (most of the other top ten collocates relate to forms of identity: 'black', 'male', 'American', 'a man', 'a woman', 'a Christian', 'a Catholic'). So I'll begin by considering some examples of 'what it means to be human'.

> Central to what it **means to be human** is God's plan for marriage and sexuality.
> What it **means to be human**: living with others before God.
> We can define what it **means to be human** by comparing the genomes.
> Biomedical advances such as cloning, challenge our understanding of what it **means to be human**.
> Biological enhancement will challenge our basic ideas about what it **means to be human**.
> What it **means to be human** is to learn to use tools to expand your abilities.

Learning gets to the heart of what it **means to be human**. Through learning we re-create ourselves.

We come to understand what it **means to be human** only within the context of our relationships.

Story form captures so much of what it **means to be human**.

Music, then, is one of the hallmarks of what it **means to be human**.

There is an almost bewildering variety of 'meanings' here. Clearly, there is not, and hardly likely to be, a consensus about 'what it means to be human', given that different voices nominate different things as fulfilling this role. Apparently, it has something to do with God's plans, the human genome, biological advances, biological enhancement, the use of tools, learning, relationships, story, and music. And that, really, is just a selection. 'What it means to be human' depends entirely on the speaker/writer's personal interests and theories, whether they be theological, genetic, anthropological, psychological, literary, or musical. Pick a theory, and read off 'what it means to be human' from that.

This is how it works. The description 'being human' is associated with an indefinitely large number of attributes. These attributes identify features that, if not always universal, are extensively distributed within our species. They range from the human genome, the hereditary information encoded in DNA; to the cultural traits studied by anthropologists – music, narrative, language, co-operation, religion, kinship structures, and so on; to personal relationships, and their psychological and sociological ramifications; to cognitive processes such as learning and problem solving; to the interaction between biology and new technology; to the stories concerning creation, transcendental forces, God's plan, or spirits, ghosts, and ancestors. To express an opinion about 'what it means to be human' is to pick out one of these features, and declare that it is the most important, or at least that it is one of a small number of attributes that have special significance.

On what basis is such a feature (or set of features) picked out? How does the speaker know that this feature represents the most important attribute, the most important predicate, out of the myriad of predicates associated with 'being human'? Well, as with all the examples of 'meaning' that we have so far considered, there is clearly a background theory, which the speaker has, and which might be shared – or possibly not – with her audience. The speaker who claims that 'Central to what it means to be human is God's plan for marriage and sexuality' obviously has a theological theory, specific to the Abrahamic monotheisms, which permits her to draw this conclusion. Some members of her audience will share this theory; others, and particularly those who have no monotheistic beliefs, will not. The speaker who suggests that 'Learning gets to the heart of what it means to be human' has a theory – it is not clear whether it is biological, psychological, or anthropological – which presumably distinguishes between the cognitive capacities of human beings and other species. Many people might agree with this claim; but all the evidence from ethological studies is that non-human animals not only learn, but also engage in problem-solving behaviour, teaching, tool use, and abstract reasoning (Russon *et al.* 1998, Pearce 2008). So, in this case, a well-informed audience might dissent from the background theory and argue that learning and using tools, in themselves, cannot be 'what it means to be human'.

This is familiar territory. 'What it means to be X' picks out an attribute, typically one of many, which is associated with X and, on the basis of a particular background theory, concludes that this attribute is of central importance. Or, to put it slightly differently: when using this construction, the speaker, on the basis of a background theory, makes an *inference* about the *salience* of a specific attribute in relation to X. So {*means + to + be*} is another construction that introduces an inference, this time an inference about the significance of an associated-with-X predicate. We can briefly consider some other examples, in order to demonstrate that this analysis does not only apply to 'What it means to be human'.

> Essentialists equate women with their vaginas, as if the vagina embodies all it **means to be** female.
> What it **means to be** feminine is to be a good mother.
> Surrendering to the what *is* of this moment: this is what it **means to be** empowered.
> What it **means to be** Jewish: to be a member of an extended family.
> The theological arithmetic of $3 = 1$ lies at the heart of what it **means to be** Christian.

These examples fit the analysis so far, with perhaps one exception. For essentialists, it is said, the most important attribute of 'being female' is the possession of a vagina. This, of all the predicates that can be assigned to femaleness, is the defining attribute, a claim supported by a biological theory of gender. An alternative inference, based on a theory that is left implicit, but which is clearly socially conservative, is that the most important predicate attached to femininity is 'being a good mother'. The most important aspect of being a Christian, according to the fifth claim, is belief in the Trinity, an inference supported by a theology that not every Christian shares. In all these examples, {*means + to + be*} represents an inference about the most salient attribute of an X, based on a theory held by the speaker, which might (or might not) be shared by her audience. So the {*means + to + be*} construction fits the general 'meaning' template.

As with earlier constructions, {*means + to + be*} is frequently used in the neutral, non-committal mode. Writers typically refer to discussions of 'what it means to be X' without taking sides, and sometimes without even specifying the candidate theories and inferences. For example:

> These movies ask us to look at what it **means to be** human.
> They must learn to negotiate an entirely new sense of what it **means to be** black.
> It is unclear just what it **means to be** male anymore.
> Millions of new immigrants are redefining what it **means to be** Christian in the US.

All these cases imply that the answer to the question 'What are the most salient attributes of being X?' is no longer clear, and that 'what it means to be X' has become problematic. Theories about the most important characteristics of X are being discussed, and it is implied that fresh answers to the question are highly likely to emerge. This sociological, non-committal, usage is the same as the one associated with {*meaning + of*}, noted earlier in the chapter.

Meaning: a summary of the analysis

I would now like to review the whole of this discussion, and offer what I take to be a general account of 'meaning' in non-lexical contexts (where we are not immediately interested in the meaning of words, the kind of meaning that can be checked in a dictionary).

The logical syntax of claims about meaning requires an inference based on some kind of theory, held by the speaker/writer. All the constructions I have considered (there are two exceptions, which I will come to in a moment) exploit this syntax, although they emphasise different parts of it and, in some cases, certain components are left implicit or unspecified. The key to understanding claims about meaning is this fundamental logic: *a theory that supports an inference.*

The logic, L, common to the {*means + that*}, {*means + participle*}, {*means + of + general concept*} and {*means + to + be*} constructions has an 'If . . . then . . .' structure. It has two versions:

L_1 If condition C holds, then, because of theory T, implication J is necessary
L_2 If condition C holds, then, because of theory T, implication J is necessary. And C holds

The 'means'/'meaning' versions of this logic are:

M_1 C means that J
M_2 C means doing J
M_3 The meaning of C is J
M_4 J is what it means to be C

It is noticeable, of course, that in the M-versions, theory T is not mentioned, which is why I have called it the background theory, and suggested that it is frequently left implicit, or at least not fully spelled out. Nevertheless, the argument I am defending is that any Meaning-statement presupposes the existence of *some* theory that is believed to justify the inference. As we have seen in many of the examples, there may be a hint about what the theory in question is; but there does not need to be. All that is required is that the speaker/writer could refer to such a theory, if requested to do so. She does not need to be able to articulate it completely, or with any degree of sophistication. The point is that the Meaning-statement is a sort of promissory note: 'There *is* a theory that supports this inference.'

Let's see how the L_1 and L_2 logic operates in some of the examples we have considered.

> If he wants a cure, then, because of physiology, giving up drugs is necessary. And he does want a cure.
>
> If meetings are only one hour per week, then, because of organisation theory, communication will be poor. And the meetings will be only one hour per week.
>
> If there is a fault in the drying cycle, then, because of the mechanism, the machine will overheat.
>
> If $a^2 - b^2 = 7$, then, because of the rules of algebra, $(a+b)\,(a-b) = 7$ can be substituted. And $a^2 - b^2 = 7$ is in fact the case.
>
> If she says it was interesting, then, because of her preference for irony, she is saying it wasn't very good. And she did say it was interesting.
>
> If a partnership is a marriage, then, because of semantics, it cannot be same-sex.
>
> If a partnership is a marriage, then, because of religious teaching, it must involve procreation.
>
> If an organism is human, then, because of biology, it must be able to use tools.
>
> If a person is feminine, then, because of [unspecified] theory, she has to be a good mother.

Notice that, in the last four, condition C refers explicitly to membership of a particular classification. In these four examples, 'If something is a member of a particular class' is a special case of 'If condition C holds'. For this reason, the inference specifies a criterion for something being a member of that class.

However, the other examples can be interpreted in the same way.

> If he is a member of the class of people who want a cure, then he must give up drugs.
>
> If the meeting is a member of the class, 'one-hour-per-week', then poor communication will result.
>
> If the drying cycle is a member of the class, 'having a fault', then the machine will overheat.
>
> If the adjective she used is a member of the class, 'interesting', then she is saying it wasn't very good.

So the differences between {*means + that*}, {*means + participle*}, {*means + of + general concept*} and {*means + to + be*} are purely marginal. The logic of the Meaning-statement is exactly the same in each case. An inference about something, classified in a certain way, depends on a background theory that applies to anything belonging to that classification.

The {*meaning + of + particular*} construction is somewhat different. The logic which applies here is L_3.

L₃   Theory T explains why condition C exists. Consequently, implication J is necessary.

With this construction, there are two Meaning-versions:

M₃   The meaning of C is J
M₅   The meaning of C is T

In other words, in this construction, the 'meaning of C' can be the explanation provided by theory T (in which case, J is implied or left unspecified). Alternatively, the 'meaning of C' can be the practical inference specified by J (in which case, theory T is implied or left unspecified). Occasionally, it is both.

This is how the analysis works out in the earlier examples:

An implicit theory T explains why there is such a thing as Christmas. Consequently, a bringing together of faith and love is necessary.

He sent Jesus to change and comfort hearts, which explains why there is such a thing as Christmas. No practical implications specified.

The birth of Christ explains why there is such a thing as Christmas. Consequently, we celebrate it with gifts.

Box 5.1 summarises the analysis, including the logical structures, the Meaning-statement equivalents, and the range of possibilities for background theory and inference. Figure 5.2 is an updated version of Figure 5.1.

Box 5.1 Formal summary

L₁   If condition C holds, then, because of theory T, J is necessary.
L₂   If condition C holds, then, because of theory T, J is necessary. And condition C holds.
L₃   Theory T explains why condition C exists. Consequently, J is necessary.

M₁   C means that J
M₂   C means doing J
M₃   The meaning of C is J
M₄   J is what it means to be C
M₅   The meaning of C is T

Theory T can be a scientific theory, a cultural or social system, a mathematical system, a language, a legal system, a theology.

Similarly, the inference J can be cause-effect, logical/mathematical, practical, or legal. Alternatively, it may clarify intention, or indicate salience.

There is a second-order, derivative use of 'the meaning of' and 'what it means to be', which refers neither to T or J, but which reports or implies, in a neutral non-committal way, that there are various theories, T₁, T₂ ... Tₙ, and various implications, J₁, J₂ ... Jₙ.

The one function that does not really fit this account is salience, at least in the form represented by the {*means + quantity noun*} construction, and two versions of the {*means + to + pronoun*} construction. In statements such as 'You really don't know how much this means to me', 'My faith means everything to me', and 'What Elvis means to me is sweet memories', the indication of salience is not an inference, as it is in {*means + to + be*}, but a simple report. The report concerns a personal response ('to me' almost always occurs in these constructions), and is clearly not based on a theory – although the speaker/writer will frequently be able to offer reasons explaining why she has that response. So, as I suggested earlier, this function is somewhat tangential. While it overlaps, to some degree, with the other salience function, {*means + to + be*}, and although the person's reasons could be regarded as analogical to the background theory implied by other constructions, it probably makes more sense to see this as an ancillary function rather than as just a variation on the basic theme of *theory-subject-inference*.

Properties, causes, experts, morality

I will discuss four matters arising. They all derive from my earlier remarks about replacing a mysterious 'realm of sense' with the linguistic function of the words 'meaning' and 'means'. Put simply, 'means' and 'meaning' are inference markers. They introduce an inference based on a theory held by the writer in question.[6] On this view, whenever somebody talks about the 'meaning of X', or 'what X means', they are presenting an inference, drawing conclusions based on a theory which they hold, but which others may well not share. (The exception is

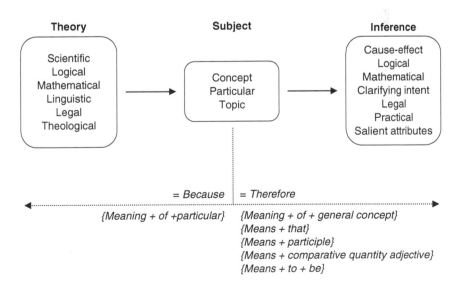

Figure 5.2 'Means' and 'meaning': updated model.

when they make a statement about salience.) If this is correct, the mystery evaporates, the metaphysical 'realms' disappear. We are talking about the theories people hold, and the inferences they base on those theories.

Here is the first comment. The picture we have of meaning is that it is a kind of *property*. If 'X means M', or 'the meaning of X is M', there is a temptation to assume that M is an attribute of X. However, on the analysis presented here, 'meaning' is *not* an attribute. It is an inference marker. In general terms:

According to A, the meaning of X is M

should be understood in the following way:

A is making an inference, M, about X, based on a theory, T

On this analysis, meaning is not in any sense a property of X; nor is it a characteristic that 'supervenes' on any property of X.[7] Instead, it is an inference-about-X proposed by A, and based on theory T. Since this inference is expressed in terms of 'means' or 'meaning', it *seems* that A is attributing a property to X (the property in question being: 'meaning M'); but this is, quite literally, a grammatical illusion.

According to A, the meaning of X is M

This sentence *looks* as if it's claiming that, according to A, something (X) has a property (M). This is because it is grammatically comparable to a sentence such as:

According to A, the colour of the cat is black

This second sentence really does claim that, according to A, something (the cat) has a property (being black). The two sentences are the same grammatically; but functionally they are quite different.

So the idea that things 'have meaning' is illusory. The business end of meaning, so to speak, is not the 'thing which has meaning' – because things don't *have* 'meanings', conceptualised as properties. On the contrary, the business end of meaning is a person who makes an inference, and the theory her inference is based on. Meaning is what an inference-maker brings to the party. It is not already 'there'. It is not, in other words, 'resident'.

Second point. Many of the theories implied in the examples I have considered are causal, to the extent that they are about X leading to Y, or Y being a consequence of X, or X making Y possible. This is nicely ironic, because meaning and cause are so frequently said to be antithetical.[8] Yet on the analysis presented here, 'meaning' turns out to be mainly a question of people's causal beliefs. The 'meanings' they 'attach' to 'phenomena' and experiences are rooted in the stories they tell about what led to what, and the explanations they offer about how things got to be where they are (Christmas, an overheated machine, fewer hunting perches for polar bears, not dying in the eternal sense). So we can't understand 'meaning' without understanding the significance of causal attributions. Meaning just *is* the causal story someone tells, and the inference she bases on it.

Exactly the same applies to the researcher. Meaning attribution is governed by her causal theories. The meaning she attributes to the phenomenon is not a property of the text, but is rooted in the theories she holds about what leads to what. Meaning just *is* the causal story she tells. Her inferences about the text, and ultimately about the phenomenon, are based on that story.

Third, if meanings are inference markers, there can be no meaning 'experts'. When Giorgi performs his meaning transformations or writes his exhaustive structures; when van Manen produces his thematic formulations and his linguistic transformations; when Benner (2000) says that humans inhabit worlds imbued with meaning, and that the goal is to discover it (Benner 1999); when de Witt *et al.* (2010) suggest that phenomenological studies provide a deeper understanding of the meaning of our everyday existence; when Fex *et al.* (2011) argue that phenomenological hermeneutical method makes possible an increased understanding by uncovering a deeper meaning of lived experiences … all these writers are signing up to the axiom of resident meaning. They are presenting themselves as experts in elucidating, unearthing, discovering, understanding, transforming, interpreting, formulating, illuminating, decoding, or uncovering meaning. The meaning they elucidate is something that awaits discovery – concealed in the text, taken for granted in the participant's account, or hidden in everyday existence – and they claim that we need scholars, phenomenologists, and hermeneutics researchers to dig it out. The truth is less metaphysical, much more prosaic. There is no resident meaning. There are only theories and inferences.

Fourth, the inferences based on causal background theories are sometimes causal themselves, but often practical, if only implicitly: because X leads to Y, one should do Z (accept compliments; keep the water troughs clean and filled; ban, or abstain from, gay marriage; display Nativity scenes at Christmas; treat everyone with the same degree of respect; remain vigilant in order to snuff out the totalitarian left's activities; be grateful to Jesus for abolishing death in the eternal sense; honour the young people who gave their lives in war; accept the Trinity; be a good mother). Some of these practical inferences are classifiable as moral injunctions: abstain from same-sex marriage; respect everyone equally; honour the young people who gave their lives; be a good mother; be grateful to God's son.

This observation echoes van Manen's (1990) claim that:

> In phenomenological research, description carries a moral force. If to be a father means to take active responsibility for a child's growth, then it is possible to say of actual cases that this or that is no way to be a father!'
>
> (12)

But there is a difference between claiming that

> the *meaning* of fatherhood [endorsed by the 'phenomenological nod'] morally obliges fathers to behave in a certain way,

and claiming that

> a particular individual has a *theory* (which others might not share), as a result of which she *believes* that fathers should do such-and-such.

Just as meaning translates into a person's inference-based-on-a-theory, so moral obligation translates into what-she-thinks-ought-to-be-done. This has a deflationary effect. The claim that 'the meaning of marriage is the union of a man and a woman, as ordained by God' must be translated into something like:

> I have this *theory* that God designed marriage to be a union of a man and a woman; accordingly, I *infer* that He does not approve of same-sex marriage, and I therefore *believe* that it should not be legalised.

Obviously, anybody who does not share the theory will be unimpressed, and will certainly not feel van Manen's 'moral force'.[9]

Method

The previous two chapters have shown that the methods adopted by Giorgi and van Manen are, at best, under-specified. For both of them, meaning is a pivotal concept; but neither provides any explanation of what it is or how to elucidate it. Nor do they suggest adequate criteria for the meaning attributions they make: the division into 'meaning units'; the identification of what is 'telling' or 'meaningful'; 'thematic formulations', 'linguistic transformations' or 'meaning transformations'; the development of 'pedagogic understandings' and the writing of 'exhaustive statements'. In the absence of such criteria, a 'meaning transformation' (in Giorgi's case) turns out to be an apparently arbitrary rewording of the original text; a 'thematic formulation' and a 'pedagogic understanding' seem to be little more than a projection of van Manen's personal values into the data.

If there are no criteria for distilling meaning from a text, then any analysis that claims to achieve this has a methodological vacuum at its centre. The gap is filled either by arbitrary changes (Giorgi), or by a particular moral view (van Manen). It's a choice between Giorgi's trivial amendments, and van Manen finding what he wants to find.

The analysis presented in this chapter explains why. Things, phenomena, experiences, data do not *have* meanings waiting to be 'unearthed' by a phenomenological expert or scholar. Meaning is not a *property* of anything. It is not resident in the text. Rather, 'means' is an inference marker. It signals the point at which the writer draws a conclusion on the basis of an antecedent theory. Meaning is what the analyst brings to the data; it is not *in* the data, awaiting discovery. Consequently, there cannot be any criteria for distilling the meaning of a phenomenon from the data, as if the data already contained it. Meaning only arrives when a theory is applied to the phenomenon concerned, and an inference is made on that basis.

Giorgi does not appear to have a theory about jealousy, and he displays a certain naivety about various psychological states. Consequently, his 'meaning analysis' creates a hodgepodge statement, combining elements of jealousy and envy. In contrast, van Manen does have theories (in particular, theories about parenting). Consequently, his 'analysis' is an unconscious projection of those theories into the data. The irony is that he presents himself as uncovering 'resident meaning' – that is, meaning already present in the data, but somehow hidden. In fact, however, he draws on antecedent theories at every stage: first, to select the 12 'left or abandoned' situations, and then to 'unearth' their 'meaning' in his 'pedagogic understanding'.

What van Manen takes himself to be doing and what he is actually doing are two different things. It is for this reason that he feels able to ascribe moral force to his phenomenological findings. He does not distinguish between two types of claim. On the one hand: 'This is the meaning of fatherhood; and it has moral force such that, if you don't behave accordingly, you are not a proper father'. On the other: 'This is my own theory of fatherhood, and I think you should behave accordingly'. His analysis warrants only the second claim; but he believes that it justifies the first.

This confusion between what is 'resident but hidden' in the data – that which must be 'uncovered' – and the inferences made by PQR researchers on the basis of antecedent theories is typical of the literature. To provide further evidence for this claim, the next chapter looks at another version of PQR developed by Smith *et al.* (2009): interpretative phenomenological analysis (IPA). This approach is insistent that interpretation, the ascription of meaning, must be 'based on a reading from within the text itself', and must not involve 'external' or 'imported' theory. However, if the analysis presented in this chapter is correct, an interpretation based exclusively on 'a reading from within the text itself' is not going to be possible.

In Chapter 6, therefore, I will consider an extended, worked-through example from Smith *et al.*'s book, and ask whether the axiom of resident meaning really does apply to it.

Notes

1 Good introductory texts on corpus linguistics include: Biber *et al.* (1998); Stubbs (2002); Teubert and Čermáková (2007); and especially McEnery and Hardie (2012).
2 Here, as throughout the book, I understand cause-and-effect as one-thing-leading-to-another-thing. As I observed in Chapter 2, note 5, those who dislike the idea of causation in human affairs usually have a very narrow concept of 'cause'.
3 An obvious question is whether it also applies to 'means' and 'meaning' in the linguistic context. Is there a connection with inferentialist semantics (Brandom 1994; Peregrin 2014)? I think there is, but it is not a direct or straightforward one, and it would be a major project to trace the connection in detail. An important stepping stone in this project would be Reiss's (2015) inferentialist reading of the meaning of causal statements.
4 The classic paper on sense and reference is Frege (1980). By far the most influential commentator on Frege's work is Dummett (1973).

5 For interesting and much more detailed accounts of how philosophers have conceptualised meaning, see: Blackburn (1984), Wettstein (2004), Medina (2005), Wilson (2006), Lee (2011), and Baz (2012).
6 Collin (1997: 217) says: 'I recommend recasting meanings as propositional attitudes'. In other words, he thinks meanings are beliefs. This is not far removed from my own analysis. However, Collin does not explore the idea that 'means' and 'meaning' are inference markers.
7 According to Azzouni (2013: 1), human beings experience physical items, products of human action, and human actions themselves, 'as having monadic meaning-properties', and do so *involuntarily*. However, this experience is an illusion since 'there are no physical objects in the world with meaning-properties of any kind. No object, that is, has the property of meaning some other thing' (5). So 'any meaning relationship between something and something else can only be one that's imposed upon these things by an experiencing person'. Obviously, I find this view congenial.
8 The idea that social science is concerned with the understanding-of-meaning not explanation-by-reference-to-cause goes back to Dilthey and Droyson, who first coined the distinction between *Erklären* (explanation) and *Verstehen* (understanding), although there are many classic statements of it (Winch 1958; von Wright 1971). In the nursing literature, Patricia Benner is probably the best known defender of this distinction (see, for example, Benner 1999).
9 There is an echo here of an interesting but neglected book by Roger Wertheimer (1972), who provides an analysis of the modal verbs, 'should', 'ought', 'must', 'can', and so on. Wertheimer is particularly interested in the moral use of 'ought', but regards this word as univocal: it means the same in 'You ought to repay the money' as it does in 'The train ought to be on time'. Obviously, I have no space for details here, but the basic idea is that any occurrence of 'ought' presupposes the existence of what Wertheimer calls a 'system' that specifies what must be true in certain conditions. This analysis covers the practical, moral, logical, and causal contexts in which 'ought' appears. The role played by a 'background theory' (according to my analysis in the text) is roughly equivalent to the role played by Wertheimer's 'system'; and I have tried to show that 'meaning' and 'means' are (more or less) univocal too, whether the inference they are used to introduce is practical, logical or causal. The verb 'to mean' is not a modal, but I think it behaves in a similar way (at least in this respect). At any rate, the similarities between Wertheimer's account of 'ought' and my account of 'means' are sufficiently marked for me to want to acknowledge them.

References

Azzouni, J. (2013) *Semantic Perception: How the Illusion of a Common Language Arises and Persists.* Oxford: Oxford University Press.

Baz, A. (2012) *When Words Are Called For: A Defense of Ordinary Language Philosophy.* Cambridge, MA: Harvard University Press.

Benner, P. (1999) 'Quality of life: a phenomenological perspective on explanation, prediction, and understanding in nursing science', in E. C. Polifroni, and M. Welch (eds.) *Perspectives on Philosophy of Science in Nursing: An Historical and Contemporary Anthology.* Philadelphia, PA: Lippincott Williams & Wilkins, pp. 303–314.

Benner, P. (2000) 'The roles of embodiment, emotion and lifeworld for rationality and agency in nursing practice', *Nursing Philosophy*, 1(1), pp. 5–19.

Biber, D., Conrad, S., and Reppen, R. (1998) *Corpus Linguistics: Investigating Language Structure and Use.* Cambridge, UK: Cambridge University Press.

Blackburn, S. (1984) *Spreading the Word: Groundings in the Philosophy of Language.* Oxford: Clarendon Press.

Brandom, R. (1994) *Making It Explicit: Reasoning, Representing and Discursive Commitment*. Cambridge, MA: Harvard University Press.

Burhans, L. M., and Alligood, M. R. (2010) 'Quality nursing care in the words of nurses', *Journal of Advanced Nursing*, 66(8), pp. 1689–1697.

Collin, F. (1997) *Social Reality*. London: Routledge.

de Witt, L., Ploeg, J., and Black, M. (2010) 'Living alone with dementia: an interpretive phenomenological study with older women', *Journal of Advanced Nursing*, 66(8), pp. 1698–1707.

Dummett, M. (1973) *Frege: Philosophy of Language*. London: Duckworth.

Fex, A., Flensner, G., Ek, A.-C., and Söderhamn, O. (2011) 'Health-illness transition among persons using advanced medical technology at home', *Scandinavian Journal of Caring Sciences*, 25(2), pp. 253–261.

Frege, G. (1980) 'On sense and reference', in P. Geach, and M. Black (eds.) *Translations form the Philosophical Writings of Gottlob Frege*. Oxford: Blackwell, pp. 56–78.

George, R. P., and Elshtain, J. B. (2006) *The Meaning of Marriage: Family, State, Market and Morals*. Dallas: Spence Publishing Company.

Hansson, K. S., Fridlund, B., Brunt, D., Hansson, B., and Rask, M. (2011) 'The meaning of the experiences of persons with chronic pain in their encounters with the health service', *Scandinavian Journal of Caring Studies*, 25, pp. 444–450.

Lee, B. (2011) *Philosophy of Language: The Key Thinkers*. London: Continuum.

McEnery, T., and Hardie, A. (2012) *Corpus Linguistics*. Cambridge, UK: Cambridge University Press.

Medina, J. (2005) *Language: Key Concepts in Philosophy*. New York: Continuum.

Murphy, M. L. (2010) *Lexical Meaning*. Cambridge, UK: Cambridge University Press.

Pearce, J. M. (2008) *Animal Learning and Cognition: An Introduction*. London: Psychology Press.

Peregrin, J. (2014) *Inferentialism: Why Rules Matter*. Basingstoke, UK: Palgrave Macmillan.

Phillips, J., and Cohen, M. Z. (2011) 'The meaning of breast cancer risk for African American women', *Journal of Nursing Scholarship*, 43(3), pp. 239–247.

Reiss, J. (2015) *Causation, Evidence, and Inference*. New York: Routledge.

Richards, J., and Bowles, C. (2012) 'The meaning of being a primary nurse preceptor for newly graduated nurses', *Journal for Nurses in Staff Development*, 28(5), pp. 208–213.

Russon, A. E., Bard, K. A., and Parker, S. T. (1998) *Reaching into Thought: The Minds of the Great Apes*. Cambridge, UK: Cambridge University Press.

Smith, J. A., Flowers, P., and Larkin, M. (2009) *Interpretative Phenomenological Analysis*. London: Sage.

Stubbs, M. (2002) *Words and Phrases: Corpus Studies of Lexical Semantics*. Oxford: Blackwell.

Swinton, J., Bain, V., Ingram, S., and Heys, S. D. (2011) 'Moving inwards, moving outwards, moving upwards: the role of spirituality during the early stages of breast cancer', *European Journal of Cancer Care*, 20(5), pp. 640–652.

Teubert, W., and Čermáková, A. (2007) *Corpus Linguistics: A Short Introduction*. London: Continuum.

Thurang, A., Fagerberg, I., Palmstierna, T., and Tops, A. B. (2010) 'Women's experiences of caring when in treatment for alcohol dependency', *Scandinavian Journal of Caring Sciences*, 24(4), pp. 700–706.

van Manen, M. (1990) *Researching Lived Experience: Human Science for an Action Sensitive Pedagogy*. Albany, NY: State University of New York Press.

von Wright, G. H. (1971) *Explanation and Understanding*. Ithaca, NY: Cornell University Press.

Wertheimer, R. (1972) *The Significance of Sense*. Ithaca, NY: Cornell University Press.

Wettstein, H. (2004) *The Magic Prism: An Essay in the Philosophy of Language*. Oxford: Oxford University Press.

Wilson, M. (2006) *Wandering Significance: An Essay on Conceptual Behaviour*. Oxford: Clarendon Press.

Winch, P. (1958) *The Idea of a Social Science*. London: Routledge and Kegan Paul.

6 Smith, Flowers, Larkin
The HIV interview

If the analysis of the previous chapter is correct, then interpretation and meaning attribution presuppose a theory of some kind. Meaning does not reside in the text, so the idea that IPA can be based exclusively on 'a reading from within the text itself' (Smith *et al.* 2009: 37), or 'a close reading of what is already in the passage' (105), has to be questioned.

The same question, of course, can be asked of any form of qualitative analysis, despite the rhetoric of 'emergent themes' (a metaphor that quietly implies that the researcher's role in this 'emergence' is minimal). Some authors do address this concern: 'When coding, are researchers active or passive? Are they merely observing patterns or meanings that "emerge" from the data, or are they actively inventing codes?' (Packer 2011: 79). My answer is that *any* code, theme, concept, comment, classification, or category adds to, and sometimes modifies, the data. By definition, it brings to the data something that does not intrinsically belong to it; and the only place this something can come from is the researcher.

SFL and theory

I will show how this works in IPA later. But first the obvious question: if SFL (Smith, Flowers and Larkin 2009) are drawing on a theory or theories in their interpretative analysis, despite all their assurances that IPA interpretation is 'tied to the text' and that theory is 'not imported from outside', what theory/theories are they employing? There are probably several implicit ones, but one of them is particularly prominent in IPA research: the idea that the 'self' and 'identity', on some understanding of those terms, are of great significance to interview respondents, especially those who have experienced a life transformation. As SFL observe: 'One of the interesting things to emerge from the growing corpus of IPA studies is how often identity becomes a central concern' (Smith *et al.* 2009: 163).

Identity and 'the self' are referred to constantly in the book's examples, and in other studies conducted by the authors and their colleagues (examples are: Flowers *et al.* 2006; Larkin and Griffiths 2002; Smith 1994, 1999; Smith and Osborn 2007). In principle, of course, there could be two possible reasons for this ubiquity. One is that identity is 'in the text', and the researcher 'finds' it there. The other is that it is projected into the text by researchers who are disposed to look for it. Obviously, SFL will argue that the first of these reasons applies. Equally obviously, given my earlier analysis, I'll argue that the second one does. A persuasive case for my view can only be made by examining SFL's examples of analysis at length and in detail, and showing that categories such as 'identity' and 'the self' cannot be derived from the data. This is what I propose to do later in the chapter. However, an example now would be useful.

One of Jonathan Smith's early studies concerned 'identity change during the transition to motherhood' (Smith 1999). Apparently, he 'had interests in identity when embarking on the project', but the construct 'took on a life of its own during the course of the study' (Smith *et al.* 2009: 163). The study concerned was longitudinal, following a small number of women through pregnancy, and exploring 'the transition to motherhood as a normative process'. In his analysis, Smith noticed 'how often the women referred to their relationships with significant others' (ibid.: 166). So at this point, he read G. H. Mead 1934), and got from him the idea that a self 'comes into being through social interaction with others.... Selves can only exist in definite relations to other selves. No hard-and-fast line can be drawn between our own selves and the selves of others' (Mead 1934: 138/164; cited in Smith *et al.* 2009: 167). As a consequence of reading Mead, there was a 'dynamic relationship' between Mead's writings and Smith's analysis of the data.

It must have been a *very* dynamic relationship. In this study, as far as I can see, there is almost nothing in the data (and there are three pages of excerpts in Smith *et al.* 2009) that warrants the comparison with Mead's ideas and concepts. Consider one of Smith's four 'theoretical statements regarding the relational self', which were 'produced through this process' (ibid.: 167):

> The symbiotic psychological relationship of self and other is facilitated and accentuated during the pregnancy by social occasions.

Two data extracts are supposed to illustrate this statement (168):

> It struck me again as I watched Paul [her partner] give his speech at the reception about the nature of all our relationships with the advent of his second family. It is important to me that Laura and Mark [Paul's children from his previous relationship] are happy and accepting and it seems that they are.
>
> (Clare)

> Thought a lot about being paranoid today. Last night Keith and I went to a friend's wedding, and I got very jealous of him talking to a friend of mine. At the time I was convinced something was going on behind my back. Today, after talking to Keith, I could see how paranoid I am. Keith forgets to tell me that I'm still attractive to him, and that I still look nice. Of course he's been fussing over me today and I feel I've been ridiculous.
>
> (Diane)

I think you have to be extremely wedded to the idea of a 'symbiotic psychological relationship of self and other' to see anything Mead-like in these extracts. Clare wants her step-children to be 'happy and accepting' (of her relationship with Paul, presumably, and the fact that she and Paul are now having a baby), and believes that they are (though there is perhaps an element of caution here: 'seems'). Diane had an experience of jealousy yesterday, which she regards as 'paranoia' today. Why this has anything to do with Mead's ontological account of the symbiotic, 'relational self' is unclear.

Okay, in Diane's case there is an implied link between her pregnancy, her anxieties about whether she is still attractive to her partner, and the jealous conviction that 'something was going on' behind her back. You can certainly suggest, on this basis, that pregnancy is changing her body, and that this is threatening to undermine a sense of her own attractiveness. You could even throw in a few 'self-' expressions: there might be a threat to her self-confidence, her self-image, her self-esteem, the sense of herself as a sexual being, and so on. But how does any of this connect to Mead? Why does it imply the idea that the 'self comes into being through social interaction with others'? How can it justify the claim that 'the symbiotic psychological relationship of self and other is facilitated and accentuated ... by social occasions'?

Equally, both women refer to family members on a social occasion. But so what? This, in itself, tells us nothing about the nature of 'selves' in general, or Clare's and Diane's 'selves' in particular. (Recall the last time you referred to your partner, your parents, or your children on a social occasion. Did that say anything about the symbiotic nature of your 'self'?) And if they believe that 'no hard-and-fast line can be drawn between our own selves and the selves of others', it is not apparent in anything they say. The only way of linking these extracts with 'symbiotic selves' is to start with Mead's concept, bring it to the analysis, find a way of hooking it up to the data, and then convince yourself it fits.

However, let's be clear about what I am *not* saying. I'm not saying Smith's interpretation is wrong. Nor am I saying that it is illegitimate to project Mead's ideas into the data. Indeed, I cannot say that, because my view is that to interpret anything involves employing a theory in order to make an inference about it. So I have no problem with Smith's use of Mead, as such. What I *am* saying is this: it's a mistake to think that the analysis 'emerges' from the data, or that it is purely 'text-driven'. Any interpretation *has* to draw on an 'imported theory' of some description. To that extent, I think SFL are kidding themselves.

It might be said that, in rejecting Smith's interpretation of the extracts from the two interviews, I must be drawing on theories of my own, even though I haven't offered an interpretation myself. Well, obviously, yes. But, again, so what? This might be an astute observation if I were arguing that drawing on theories was for some reason illegitimate. But I am, precisely, not arguing that. I am arguing that drawing on a theory is inevitable in all cases of meaning attribution. It goes with the territory. Later, when I examine SFL's example, I will specify what theories I employ in rejecting SFL's interpretation, and in offering my own. The difference between SFL and me will turn out to be: (a) we have different theories, (b) they think the analysis, or at least the first stage of it, can be external-theory-free. They think that the meaning they attribute to the data is resident in the text. I think they're mistaken.

Reading the IPA corpus creates the distinct impression that Smith's encounter with Mead, and the way in which this encounter encouraged him to embrace the 'self' and 'identity' vocabulary, set an agenda for subsequent IPA studies. It is not just the fact that so many of these studies set out to examine the consequences for 'identity' of illness-related life-transitions. Nor is it just the fact that IPA researchers are primed to link their data with 'identity' themes during analysis. It is also that they may unwittingly attempt to elicit 'identity-friendly' material during the interview. We will see an example of this later.

Theory and classification

Self-consciously intellectual (if vague) concepts such as 'identity' and 'the self' are obvious indicators of theory-dependent interpretation. However, qualitative analysis incorporates other analytical routines that are equally theory-dependent, though in a much less transparent manner. There is a spectrum of procedures in which theory-dependence can be seen, ranging from Smith's 'dynamic relationship' to the most basic of analytical steps, such as coding and classification.

Almost all types of qualitative analysis involve classification. This is most obviously true of those that involve attaching labels (that is, 'codes') to segments of data; or assigning several segments to the same category; or assembling categories into themes. However, it is also (though perhaps less obviously) true of those that emphasise meaning attribution. In all cases, a segment of data is brought under a heading, and thereby grouped with other segments: from the same transcript, the same study, or any other context in which the word or phrase used to specify the category might occur. This grouping both includes and excludes. It identifies the segment with others brought under the same heading; and it differentiates them from those to which that heading has not been applied.

Where do these groups and headings come from? Typically, methodological texts are vague about this. Often, there is some reference to a search for 'underlying uniformities and diversities' (Glaser and Strauss 1967: 114); 'similar words and phrases, used to express the same idea' (Auerbach and Silverstein 2003: 37); 'units of information with similar content' (Teddlie and Tashakkori 2009: 253); 'similarities and differences' (Kvale and Brinkman 2009: 202); or 'similar meanings' (Holloway and Wheeler 2010: 287).

The problem should be obvious. 'Similar' in what way? The 'same' in what respect? Similarity does not, by itself, define a relation. Imagine being in a large room full of people and being asked to point to two of them who are 'the same' or 'similar'. The question barely makes sense. Similar in age, gender, height, build, colour of eyes, dress, ethnicity, first language, position in their respective families, location in the room, birthday...? Without a *criterion* of some kind, whether explicit or implied, identifying two people who are the 'same' is just not possible. If you pick out two anyway, the choice will either be arbitrary, or determined (consciously or unconsciously) by a criterion of your own. In any case, the criterion will not be 'emergent' from the group of people themselves.

The invitation to identify 'units of information with similar content' is of a comparable kind. However, in research practice it is often difficult to see this because we are so used to the 'coding and categorising' routine that the problem slides by unnoticed.[1] Smith's analysis of 'identity change during the transition to motherhood' study again provides an example.

Smith considers a long extract from Diane's research diary in which several episodes involving herself, her partner Keith, and her eight-year-old brother David are described. In the first, David asks whether she and Keith will be getting married before or after her baby is born. Keith asks him whether he thinks it makes any difference, and David shrugs his shoulders. 'But it made me think whether the baby would worry about it when he or she grew up.' In the second, Keith and David are drilling the concrete out in the hallway, when Diane bangs her head on the stairs and starts 'crying like a baby'. Keith comforts her, and checks for a cut. 'Any other time I would have just sworn, rubbed my head and gone on. I don't know whether I was just tired or after a bit of attention.' In the third, Diane is making a clown mobile for the baby's room. Keith has taken David to the pub garden to play. Keith and David arrive home, and Diane goes to check the dinner. While she is out of the room, Keith

> cut the hat so that it fits the clown's head. I went mad, and screamed at him for touching my belongings. I said 'what's the point of teaching children not to touch other people's belongings if even he can't do it'. Keith was astounded by my reaction and laughed at me. But I felt quite angry about it.
>
> (169)

The extract is used to illustrate another of the four 'theoretical statements regarding the relational self':

> The increasing psychological engagement with significant others during pregnancy can facilitate the psychological preparation for mothering.

Here is how Smith interprets Diane's journal entries:

> Notice how individuals' family roles change within the extract. It begins with Keith playing an adult role and Diane being like a child. In the third [exchange], Keith plays 'father' to David's 'child' but then, in a sense, seems to regress to himself being a child scolded by Diane or 'the mother', after which he is transformed to the world parent again.
>
> So the roles are quickly interchangeable. Diane is baby and mother, Keith is carer, child and cynical adult, all within the space of one episode. Perhaps Diane is here psychologically exploring these different family roles, and particularly what it means to be a child, from a number of different

perspectives and it is the symbiotic connection of self concept with conception of others which allows this to happen.

(170)

Smith is arguing that the three episodes are 'units of information with similar
content'. They can be placed in a single category referring to adult/parent/child
roles, and show how these roles are swapped between Diane and Keith. The
'theoretical statement' implies that this process is part of psychological preparation for mothering. To persuade us of this, he has to suggest that, at different
times, 'Diane is baby and mother', while 'Keith is carer, child and cynical adult'.
But to persuade us of *that*, he has to portray Keith's reaction to Diane's anger
(about the clown mobile) as a 'regression to himself being a child scolded by the
mother'. (He also has to justify the description of Keith as a 'cynical adult'. I
have no idea where this description comes from.)

I can see absolutely nothing in Diane's account to warrant this. 'Keith was
astounded by my reaction and laughed at me.' How on earth does that sentence
merit the description 'Keith regressing to himself being a child scolded by the
mother'? Aside from the irony of Smith's implicit appeal to psychoanalytic
theory (regression), there is a considerable leap from this data segment to how
Smith wants to classify it

There is a case for saying that Diane takes on the child role when she 'cries
like a baby'. But even if we agree to that description, it is still a stretch to portray
this as some sort of 'psychological preparation for motherhood'. It is at least
equally plausible to portray it as a result of emotional fragility consequent on her
pregnancy. (Indeed, on my reading, there are several examples of her emotionally labile reactions in the extracts from this study.)

As for Diane exploring 'what it means to be a child from a number of different perspectives', you could perhaps argue that the first episode – wondering
whether the baby will worry about her parents' marital status later in life – fits
this description. But is Smith seriously suggesting that banging her head, crying,
and getting very angry ('I went mad') because Keith has touched the clown
mobile can be placed in the same category? Well, apparently he is. Equally
unexpectedly, he is also suggesting that this 'exploring' is made possible by 'the
symbiotic connection of self concept with conception of others'. I don't think
there is any sense in which this can be derived from the data, with or
without Mead.

So Smith's attempt to place these three data segments in the same category –
to represent them as 'units of information with similar content' – requires a lot
of special pleading. The category certainly does not 'emerge' from the text, and
is not even 'closely tied' to it. Keith 'regressing' and Keith as 'cynical adult' just
do not map on to the data. Neither, really, does Diane 'exploring what it means
to be a child'. There is no prospect of justifying the 'adult/parent/child roles' category without imported theory ('regression'), without distorting the data, and
without skating round a number of inconvenient features of the text that
don't fit.[2]

A quick reminder of what I said earlier. I am *not* arguing that Smith is wrong to create this category, or that it is illegitimate to import theories (from whatever source). I *am* arguing that the category is theory-dependent, and that it cannot be derived exclusively from the data.

My theory, which is mine[3]

In the second half of this chapter, I will examine an extended example of IPA, as presented by SFL, and contrast my interpretation with theirs. To prepare the ground for that, I must first specify the theories I will be drawing on. They fall into three groups: theories about psychological mechanisms; theories about the interview process; and theories about language use. Here, I only summarise the relevant theories, and will make no attempt to evidence them.

Psychological mechanisms

As a default, people do not understand their own motivation. We do not have introspective access to the causes of our own behaviour (though we can infer them by observing our behaviour and by registering sensory input, whether from the environment or from our own bodies). Ordinarily, people do not need access to their motives, since most daily life consists in just getting on with stuff. But, when asked to explain their actions, people standardly offer a theory drawn from a culturally available repertoire (the 'vocabulary of motive'), a theory that provides an explanation of that *type* of action in that *type* of circumstance. Such an account may be true (or not) in the particular case; however, it is derived from the repertoire, and not from privileged access to something 'inside' the person concerned. (Sources for these ideas include: Nisbett and Wilson 1977; Heidegger 1962; Mills 1940; Wilson 2002; Hassin *et al.* 2005).

There is, at best, an indeterminacy about some psychological states, such as emotions and desires, which are two-dimensional vectors rather than discrete points in a multi-dimensional psychological space. For example, an emotion has two axes: valence (positive or negative) and the degree of arousal. But how the emotion is described, specifically, depends on contextual factors. Someone can be aware of a 'negative' form of arousal, and be able to recognise it as mild, moderate or intense. But whether it is described as 'fear', 'anger', 'hatred', 'disgust' or 'jealousy', will depend on the circumstances in which it is aroused. Equally, how it is described later, when the person concerned looks back over a period of weeks, months or years, depends on the way in which those circumstances are retrospectively conceptualised (Feldman Barrett 2006; Carruthers 2011; Schwitzgebel 2011; Vazire and Wilson 2012).

In general, our actions, intentions, emotions, preferences, desires, and motives are governed by a range of psychological mechanisms of which we are rarely conscious, and to which we have no 'inner' access. Many of these mechanisms take the form of cognitive biases, such as the fundamental attribution error, social desirability bias, self-serving bias, the framing effect, availability bias, and hindsight bias. Other mechanisms include: cognitive dissonance, priming, anchoring, imitation (Kunda 1999; Hassin *et al.* 2005; Kahneman 2011; Doris 2015).

The interview

The interview is an example of social interaction. No qualitative researcher would dispute this claim in principle, but it is routinely ignored in practice. In such a highly social species as our own, every detail of the social exchange between two people is potentially significant, with both parties examining what the other person says, for material that will provide clues as to their respective social standing, what is expected of them, the extent to which they fulfil their obligations, and the most effective strategies for avoiding embarrassment. This is particularly true of the respondent, since she is present at the invitation of the interviewer, and is likely to be less clear about the status and function of the exchange itself. This social evaluation is largely subconscious, but among its consequences are the following: as a default, the respondent will be anxious to please (or not displease) the interviewer; both sides, but especially the participant, will be concerned to present themselves in a certain light, and as a certain kind of person; and the participant's responses will be highly sensitive to what the interviewer says – how questions are phrased, how they are ordered, and how the interviewer reacts to answers, and so on (Rapley 2001; Sabini *et al.* 2001; Potter and Hepburn 2005; Zawidzki 2013).

One critical parameter of the interview is the respondent's understanding of the task, not only in general terms but in relation to each question. All things being equal, one might expect the interviewer to make this as clear as possible by specifying precisely the information being requested. However, there is a counter-imperative in some forms of qualitative research, including PQR, which discourages questions that incorporate the researcher's own categories. This counter-imperative implies, not precise questions, but vague, 'open-ended' ones which don't give the respondent much to go on. It is as if the participant were invited to 'talk about it in the way you would have talked about it if you hadn't been asked to talk about it'. In practice, though, this doesn't matter much because, typically, the interviewer's reactions to the participant's responses – welcoming or otherwise – will provide the necessary clues. In this way, the interviewer can claim to respect the respondent's calibrations while subtly, or not so subtly, imposing her own. This often involves coaching the respondent in the relevant research agenda (Antaki and Rapley 1996; Potter and Hepburn 2005; Baker 2001; van den Berg *et al.* 2003).

In both the conduct of interviews and in subsequent data analysis, PQR researchers generally assume that the respondent is a reliable guide to her own psychological states. However, as I suggested above, respondents cannot be regarded as authorities on either 'inner states' or 'inner causal processes'. Indeed, the function of the respondent's talk about psychological states and processes is not to describe 'internal goings-on'. Rather, it is to accomplish social rather than epistemic goals: for example, to get along with the interviewer; to elicit sympathy or admiration; to fulfil a responsibility; to rationalise or excuse past behaviour; to present the respondent as somebody who meets a culturally prescribed norm ... and so on. (Mills 1940; Edwards 1997; Myers 2004; Zawidzki 2013).

Language use

The utterances that people produce during conversation – and, as most qualitative researchers insist, the interview is one form of conversation – can only be understood in context. This is another maxim that is universally recognised in principle but frequently overlooked in practice, especially when 'context' is taken to include what Sinclair (1997: 34) calls 'co-text'; that is, the immediate verbal environment of the interview itself. For this is a conversation of an unusual type, one in which many of the familiar rules of conversational relevance are suspended, or at least modified. Or so it can seem to the respondent, who commonly tries to apply these rules, but finds that they have to be renegotiated *in situ*. The participant's utterances are a response to the interviewer, not in the sense of being answers to a series of questions, but as attempts to decode the conversation's relevance assumptions. The interview can be construed, in part, as a social process in which the relevant contextual assumptions have to be created, negotiated and defined during the course of the conversation itself (Grice 1991; Sinclair 1997; Sperber and Wilson 1995; Widdowson 2004).

From another perspective, the interview transcript can be considered as a document, independently of the social processes that produced it. Like other documents – for example, newspaper articles, blogs, or song lyrics – it has a content with a certain distribution. Some topics get greater attention, others get less. Some items are couched in positive terms, others in negative terms. Some claims are made without restriction, others are hedged with epistemic qualifiers ('I believe', 'I suppose', 'I think', 'perhaps'). It is reasonable to assume that these distributions are salient to the respondent. All things being equal, topics to which more space is devoted are of greater significance to her; positive and negative framings indicate valence; epistemic qualifiers are symptoms of hesitation, doubt, ignorance, or uncertainty. Quantitative content analysis is designed to identify and measure these distributions. Although it has most commonly been applied to samples of media texts, it can also be applied to a single document such as an interview transcript, in order to determine the salience attached to various topics by the respondent. This affords a more checkable criterion of salience than picking out 'key words' or 'significant statements', which is what PQR authors propose (Weber 1990; Wierzbicka 2006; Krippendorff 2013; Riffe *et al.* 2013).

The HIV interview

The rest of this chapter is devoted to an examination of SFL's most extensive example, the analysis of an excerpt from an interview transcript. The respondent is Jack, a man in his mid-twenties who was invited to talk about his experiences of living with HIV (he was diagnosed in his early twenties). The details of the analysis are presented on pages 85–88 and 93–95, although there is a theoretical commentary throughout the chapter.

Box 6.1 reproduces the interview excerpt in full, as it appears in the book.

Box 6.1 The HIV interview

I: Are you alright to tell me more about that?

R: More about that um ... don't know if it was, hm ... I think that was really because I had, I just I just didn't know who ... in lots of ways I didn't know who I was, at that time, in the early days of being diagnosed and coming to terms with it, I couldn't stop thinking about it and um ... I had to go through a process of finding out or finding myself again, um, and whilst I was around people that knew me well well, I found it really really exhausting because, well well maybe they couldn't tell but I was sure, I was paranoid that that they would know that something was wrong, so I was constantly trying to to be as near to how I imagined myself to being without HIV so ... that in itself made it even more impossible, because the more you try to stop thinking about something, then the harder it becomes, you know so...

I: And then, these these are your close friends are you thinking about?

R: Close friends, family, anybody, even new people that I'd meet; I just felt that I couldn't, I suppose I felt quite quite worthless because I didn't have the [sighs] I felt like I'd lost something I couldn't um ... I just found everything so tiring, I couldn't, I didn't have anything to give, I didn't feel that I had anything worthwhile to kind of contribute or you know, the, I don't know, I was just kind of like shell-shocked I supposed, you know. [sorry] So ... I don't know if that's answered the...

I: Are you up, do you see the kind of style of questions that? [yeah yeah] And again you just, you said some amazing things about a sense of loss, a sense of being worthless or nothing being worthwhile. But ... and are you alright with talking [yeah yeah] [unclear] but what would you say that you had lost?

R: Ju just er ... what had I lost? Um ... I'd lost the feeling that I had all the time in the world kind of, that I'd um ... I'd realised that at some point I was going to die, whether that was going to be 15, 20 how ever many years, I'd realised that that could happen and er ... I think that's what I'd lost. Um ... but also I'd lost my self esteem and my self respect as well because, I'm not sure why um, well because of the relationship that I was in but also because of the diagnosis definitely um ... it was a big big part of it.

The interview process

I have a few comments to make on this excerpt before looking at the details of SFL's analysis. First, the interviewer appears to adopt the minimalist approach, complying with the counter-imperative (as I called it earlier) which discourages questions incorporating the researcher's own categories. S/he does manage to produce a specific question ('What would you say that you had lost?')

eventually, but for the rest s/he does not really give the respondent any clues about what s/he wants to know, and why. It is interesting to contrast this with an interview excerpt from another textbook (Buunk and Van Vugt 2013: 63–64), in which the respondent is a female employee who refused to accept a management position at her company.

FEMALE EMPLOYEE: I didn't want the job.
SOCIAL PSYCHOLOGIST: Why not?
FEMALE EMPLOYEE: I didn't feel it was the right job for me.
SOCIAL PSYCHOLOGIST: Why wasn't it right for you?
FEMALE EMPLOYEE: I don't like to tell other people what to do.
SOCIAL PSYCHOLOGIST: What is it about that that you don't like?
FEMALE EMPLOYEE: I don't think they would listen to me.
SOCIAL PSYCHOLOGIST: Why do you think that?
FEMALE EMPLOYEE: Maybe because most of them are men and they don't take women managers very seriously.
SOCIAL PSYCHOLOGIST: What makes you think that? Can you give examples?
FEMALE EMPLOYEE: There haven't been any female managers and the one who was briefly here left the job after less than a year.
SOCIAL PSYCHOLOGIST: Why do you think that is?
FEMALE EMPLOYEE: Because she couldn't get along with her staff.
SOCIAL PSYCHOLOGIST: What types of problem did she have with her staff?
FEMALE EMPLOYEE: Her staff thought that the only reason she got the job was because of an affirmative action programme.
SOCIAL PSYCHOLOGIST: And was this true, do you think?
FEMALE EMPLOYEE: No, but I don't think the top management in the company did enough to support her.
SOCIAL PSYCHOLOGIST: What makes you think that?
FEMALE EMPLOYEE: Hm … maybe they thought that helping her would give out the wrong signal.
SOCIAL PSYCHOLOGIST: What kind of wrong signal?
FEMALE EMPLOYEE: Perhaps they were afraid that it would undermine her authority if they offered help.

The contrast between this and the SFL example could hardly be more stark. Buunk and Van Vugt concede that the questions posed by the psychologist 'are a bit unimaginative'; and it is true that the questioning process could have been considerably less ritualistic and staccato. But every question is specific, leaving the respondent in no doubt as to what information is being sought; and the interviewer single-mindedly pursues a line of thought, seeking to dig out at every opportunity the reasons for the previous answer.

In contrast, the SFL interviewer makes no more than vague gestures, and the respondent has to make do with only sketchy indications of what is being asked, at least initially. To a considerable extent, I think, this explains his hesitancy, his uncertainty, and the fact that he jumps from one topic to another without warning. If you have no idea what the interviewer wants to know, this is something you tend to do.

For example, the interviewer begins the excerpt with 'Are you alright to tell me more about that?' This is content-depleted in the sense that the respondent can have little or no clue about what kind of 'more' the interviewer is looking for. Consequently, he spends the next four lines hunting for a suitable topic that might fit: 'don't know if it was...', 'didn't know who I was', 'coming to terms with it', 'couldn't stop thinking about it', 'finding myself again'. Each of these represents a distinctly different line of thought, which the interviewer could have asked specific questions about. Finally, however, Jack homes in on the business of pretending to his friends and family that nothing was wrong, and how difficult and exhausting that was.

Instead of picking up on any of these topics, and pursuing them in the manner of Buunk and Van Vugt, the SFL interviewer says: 'And then, these ... are your close friends are you thinking about?' Perhaps unsurprisingly, this produces another somewhat meandering response, which ranges over being shocked, losing something, everything being tiring, not having anything to give, and so on.

Again, any of these could have been the trigger for a series of specific, information-yielding, questions; and, this time, the interviewer does in fact pick out one topic in particular. However, s/he gives it a special twist: 'you said some amazing things about a sense of loss, a sense of being worthless or nothing being worthwhile'. This, finally, gives the respondent a clear indication of what the interviewer regards as important – above all else, I'm tempted to add – by cuing him with 'amazing'.

It is this 'amazing' topic that will be welcomed, indeed applauded, by the interviewer, so naturally the respondent goes for it. Initially, he suggests that he has potentially lost years off his life. This is what he appears to emphasise, in fact ('I think that's what I'd lost'). But after a pause ('Um'), he recalls that the interviewer was particularly taken with 'being worthless' and 'nothing being worthwhile', so he throws in loss of self-esteem for good measure. At first, he attributes this loss of self-esteem to his relationship, but then realises (as it seems) that this is slightly off-message, so he attributes it additionally ('definitely um') to the diagnosis.

On my reading, therefore, the interviewer gives the respondent very little to go on, as a result of which he stumbles around different aspects of the experience. Finally, he mentions loss and feeling worthless; and at this point the interviewer cues him with 'you said some amazing things'. This transparent 'let's-have-some-more-of-that' signal is successful, in that the respondent takes the cue, and develops the loss and feeling worthless theme. A topic that was originally one among others, with no particular emphasis placed on it, has been amplified into the central theme of the interview.

It is hard to avoid the suspicion that the interviewer was looking for the self-loss-worthless cluster, cued it, and then amplified it. If so, it is not surprising that it figures so prominently in the subsequent analysis – partly because it is endemic to the SFL analytical agenda, and partly because it is genuinely thematic in the interview (because it has been cued and amplified by the interviewer). The circularity here should be evident (Figure 6.1).

The reader, or indeed SFL, might dispute my interpretation. I have, after all, implicitly ascribed various thoughts to the respondent in my comments above. Is this not unduly speculative? Certainly it is. But so what? In the first place, I have been no more speculative than SFL are in their own analysis (as we shall see in a moment). In the second place, the SFL approach is *interpretive*. This is my interpretation. If it is disputed, on what grounds? Why are my speculations inferior to, or less plausible than, SFL's? It is true that we are using different theories to 'make sense' of what the respondent says. But that is precisely the point.

The structure of the analysis

The analysis characteristic of IPA is presented as consisting of six steps, although SFL suggest that this is to 'minimize the potential for the novice analyst's anxiety and confusion' (81), and that it should not be understood as a recipe. The six steps are: [1] reading and re-reading; [2] initial noting; [3] developing emergent themes; [4] searching for connections across emergent themes; [5] moving to the next case; [6] looking for patterns across cases. The chapter includes another section entitled 'Taking it deeper: levels of interpretation', which is effectively a seventh step. Here, I will focus primarily on step [2], since this is where the action is.

Step [2] is, according to SFL, the most detailed and time consuming. It 'examines semantic content and language use on a very exploratory level' (83). For the sake of illustration, exploratory commenting is 'broken down into three discrete processes with different focuses'. These are (84):

> *Descriptive* comments focused on describing the content of what the participant has said
> *Linguistic* comments focused on exploring the specific use of language by the participant
> *Conceptual* comments focused on engaging at a more interrogative and conceptual level

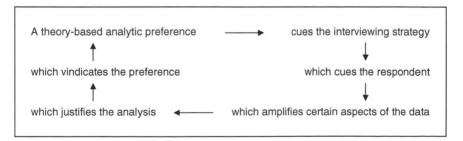

Figure 6.1 The circularity of the HIV interview.

In the book, and in the analysis as reproduced below, the following key is used:

> Descriptive comments = normal text
> Linguistic comments = *italic*
> Conceptual comments = underlined

I will go through the interview line by line, appending SFL's comments on each part of the respondent's text (both indented). However, I will also add my own interpretation (remarking on SFL's interpretation, by way of contrast). Effectively, two different readings of the transcript are provided: SFL's and mine. They tell two different stories, drawing on the different theories that SFL and I bring to the data. In my own case, the relevant theories were summarised above. The key point remains that *no* interpretation can be based on the data alone.

The transcript includes three 'speeches' made by Jack, in answer to the interviewer's promptings. I've given each speech a separate section. There is a summary at the end.

First speech

The interviewer's question is: 'Are you alright to tell me more about that?' I have already suggested that this does not give Jack much to go on, because the interviewer does not specify what kind of 'more' s/he has in mind. S/he gives no indication of what s/he wants to know, or why. Unsurprisingly, Jack's initial response is tentative and uncertain.

> More about that um … don't know if it was, hm … I think that was really because I had, I just

> *Is there an underlying difficulty in articulating something this emotive and complex [repetition of 'I' and 'to']? Clear sense of struggling to articulate something very strong and confusing difficult feelings. Use of 'just' emphasizes his struggle to explain.*

After the interviewer's minimalist question, Jack responds with a series of stops-and-starts, having no idea what's wanted. These are, at best, half thoughts, begun then interrupted as he casts around for a suitable and coherent line of thought. However, SFL attempt to find something 'emotive', 'complex', 'strong', 'confusing', and 'difficult' in Jack's mundane stumbling.

> I just didn't know who … in lots of ways I didn't know who I was,

> Major issue of questioning self. Who is Jack? Many ways in which self-questioning occurred. Who are you if you're not yourself? Diagnosis and self-questioning are clearly linked? Impact of diagnosis

More of the same. The only reason for thinking that this has special significance, or that it has anything to do with the 'self', is because SFL say it has. Look at it in the context of what precedes and follows it, and it becomes just another bit of stumbling talk, picking up then putting down a particular idea from a range of possible topics. Jack is still looking for clues as to what he's supposed to talk about.

> At that time, in the early days of being diagnosed and coming to terms with it, I couldn't stop thinking about it and um...

Critical sense of time frame (these experiences are embedded within time, has he come to terms with it now?) Maybe ideas like stages or vulnerable periods? Overwhelmed with thinking about HIV

Another change of gear. There is no connection between 'I didn't know who I was', which immediately precedes it, and 'I couldn't stop thinking about it'. The passage is characterised by a series of topic shifts, which occur every dozen words or so. However, SFL make another attempt to project conceptual depth into this passage: a 'critical sense of time frame', 'embedded experiences', 'stages'. This clearly exceeds what the respondent says.

> I had to go through a process of finding out

If something was found what was lost? Who does the finding in finding themselves?

Again, the thought starts and stops. There is no clue here as to how this fragment might continue if the thought were pursued further. SFL want to link it with the next bit, because of the repetition of *finding*. But that is the *only* reason for thinking there is a connection, and it is pretty thin. Of course, if you are disposed to latch on to anything that can be framed as having something to do with the 'self', then you might put this fragment and the next together, and suggest that the idea of losing and finding oneself is thematic to the whole extract. However, until the interviewer's interest is signalled by 'amazing things', it is just one small part of Jack's stumbling around.

In any case, SFL's question 'If something was found what was lost?' is puzzling, because 'find out' (as opposed to 'find') is a synonym of 'discover' or 'learn'. It does not imply that anything has been lost. In this context, Jack could be talking about the implications, causes or management of his condition. 'I had to go through a process of finding out ... [about HIV]'. Or: 'I had to go through a process of finding out how best to deal with the fact that I couldn't stop thinking about it'. Given the passage that precedes it, this is more plausible than SFL's reading.

> Or finding myself again, um,

Impact of diagnosis. Does diagnosis mean you lose yourself?

This, of course, is IPA gold. Finding myself. Losing myself. The self. This figures prominently among the 'emergent themes' in step [3]: 'The questioning self', 'Lost self', and 'Finding the self (process)'. But that is an awful lot to hang on remarkably few words. Suppose we add together the two phrases that allegedly support this 'emergent theme': namely, 'finding myself again' and 'I didn't know who I was'. That makes a grand total of nine words referring to the idea that SFL make so much of. And that is nine words out of the 165 words in Jack's first speech. The 'self' is an emergent theme only because SFL want it to be.

> And whilst I was around people that knew me well well, I found it really really exhausting because, well well maybe they couldn't tell but I was sure, I was paranoid that that they would know that something was wrong, so I was constantly trying to to be as near to how I imagined myself to being without HIV so...

Importance of people who knew him. <u>What does this say for the importance of social context? Is the self social?</u>
Emphasizing the enormity of the task with repetition of 'really'
Found it exhausting
Hesitant repetitions (well, well and I, I)
<u>Is paranoia an over concern with others' view of self?</u>
'Wrong', the old self was 'right'? Performance. Working to manage people's perceptions of himself. Some sense of performing, some pivotal loss of authenticity implicit within this, how can you perform yourself? Who is doing the performance? How can a medical procedure lead to this radical sense of being lost?
Tails off.

And it's gone again. 'Finding myself' turns out to be yet another half thought, another brief fragment, that Jack picks up and then immediately puts down. Instead of developing it, he turns to a wholly new idea, one to which he has not so far referred. This is the observation that he found it really exhausting to pretend to his friends that nothing was wrong. At 60 words, this is the first idea to be elaborated beyond 25 words, and only one of two that is elaborated beyond 12 (the other is: '...at that time ... I couldn't stop thinking about it...'). Both passages have a *prima facie* claim to salience.

As for SFL's comments. 'What does this say for the importance of social context? Is the self social?' On what basis can you infer this from what Jack says, unless you are on a Mead-hunting expedition? Does *any* reference to what other people are thinking imply that 'selves can only exist in definite relations to to other selves'? How would you justify that claim? Jack misuses the term 'paranoia', as most of us do colloquially. He means that he was chronically anxious that people would know something was wrong. SFL's attempt to make something more of this is Mead-motivated. ' "Wrong", the old self was "right"?' This again twists the text beyond recognition. Jack was afraid people would know something was wrong – in other words, that he had been diagnosed with a life-limiting illness. Only someone who is already theoretically committed would turn this into a question about his 'self'. I don't have a problem with the idea of 'performing' in this context. But the question 'How can you perform yourself? Who is doing the performance?' is silly. SFL are straining to find philosophical significance in every mundane, colloquial thing Jack says.

> That in itself made it even more impossible, because the more you try to stop thinking about something, then the harder it becomes, you know so...

Things were impossible
Internal thinking about himself
Intra-psychic process implied, thinking about thinking, major change in sense of his own mind. Impact of diagnosis. Does diagnosis make you think about thinking? Think about self?

Although he doesn't spell it out, Jack is presumably referring to the diagnosis when he talks about trying to stop thinking about something. Earlier, he said: 'I couldn't stop thinking about it'. Here, he implies that he was *trying* to stop thinking about it. The idea is a familiar one: it can be virtually impossible to stop thinking about something if you are trying *not* to think about it. In fact, as Jack seems to say here, it may be that trying not to think about it just makes you think about it more. In pretending to his friends that nothing was wrong, Jack was 'trying to to be as near to how I imagined myself to being without HIV'. This would presumably mean inhibiting any thoughts about 'himself *with* HIV'; and that clearly implies trying not to think about the diagnosis. So not being able to stop thinking about it might be an effect of trying to stop thinking about it, which might partly be a consequence of pretending to his friends that everything was okay (because that required imagining himself without HIV). If all of that is correct, it's no wonder he found it exhausting.

Three further comments before I move on to Jack's next speech. First, if the section from 'whilst I was around...' to '...becomes, you know so' does represent a single line of thought, however incompletely expressed, then 88 of the 165 words in this speech are on that topic. Indeed, if we add 'at that time, in the early days of being diagnosed and coming to terms with it, I couldn't stop thinking about it', which looks as if it is referring to the same basic idea, that makes 110 words out of 165 devoted to this theme. According to my take on content analysis, that counts as highly salient. In contrast, for SFL to fasten on the 'finding myself' references – nine words out of 165 – and propose that 'losing and finding oneself' is a crucial part of Jack's thinking is a trifle forced.

Second, the line of thought in question is actually rather interesting. It raises some intriguing questions about the psychology of a diagnosis such as HIV. Why, for example, does Jack try to pretend nothing was wrong? Given that he does, exactly what strategies does he pursue in trying to make the pretence

convincing? Am I right in supposing that 'trying to to be as near to how I imagined myself to being without HIV' requires an effort not to think about the
diagnosis? If I am, how does that work? What cognitive strategies does Jack
employ to achieve this? If I'm not right, what *does* it require? How did he set
about the task of being 'near to how I imagine myself being without HIV'? He
does, of course, make some gestures towards explaining his strategy, but they
are rather vague and he does not articulate his thoughts very well. In view of
this, the interviewer could have put some of these questions to him.

Third, I can't see anything in the text to justify SFL's reference to 'major
change in sense of his own mind'. Jack is expressing a familiar idea – that *not*
thinking about something that makes you anxious is almost impossible. So the
question 'Does diagnosis make you think about thinking?' misses the point.
Meanwhile, 'Think about self?' is a transparent effort to find another peg to hang
the 'self' on.

Second speech

The interviewer says: 'And then, these these are your close friends are you thinking about?' Well, this is something that can be picked out of the first speech, but
it's not clear why the interviewer latches on to it, given that there are other interesting avenues to explore.

> Close friends, family, anybody, even new people that I'd meet;

> Everyone knew
> Begins with sense of people who knew the 'old' Jack but then includes 'new'
> people. Centrality of others and their thinking about him (all in absence of
> knowing his status too). It's all in his mind if he hasn't disclosed.

SFL's descriptive comment 'Everyone knew' is baffling. Jack has said that he
worried that people who knew him well would realise that something was
wrong, and that while he was around them he 'found it really really exhausting'.
It is evident that he was pretending nothing was wrong with everybody, 'even
new people that I'd meet', as he admits here; but the anxiety that people might
see through the pretence was particularly strong with those who knew him best.
This makes sense, of course. It is likely that the pretence was particularly
exhausting (and perhaps not as successful) around close friends, who would be
more likely to recognise that he was hiding something; a new acquaintance
would hardly know him well enough to tell. In view of this, it is impossible to
see why SFL think that the comment 'Everyone knew' is appropriate.

> I just felt that I couldn't,

It is by no means clear what this refers to. Couldn't what? The SFL analysis
appears to link it with the next bit, but there is no obvious reason to do so. It is

more likely that Jack is following a train of thought connected with the exhausting business of pretending that everything is fine. Recall that he has just said: **'that in itself made it even more impossible, because the more you try to stop thinking about something, then the harder it becomes, you know so...'** In this context, it is more likely – it is certainly no less likely – that he was heading in the direction of: 'I just felt that I couldn't keep up the pretence, because it was so draining.'

I suppose I felt quite quite worthless because I didn't have the [sighs]

He felt worthless. *Repetition of 'I' and 'quite', emphasizing meaning*
Sighs (sharing grief?) He had lost something

Of course, *worthless* will immediately attract the interviewer's attention – it is an idea s/he is primed for by the SFL approach – and s/he will connect it, in a moment, to the sense of loss. But let's look at this sentence in the context in which it occurs. Jack is talking about pretending to his friends that nothing is wrong, and about how exhausting that is. Notice that, on the next line, he repeats this idea: **'I just found everything so tiring'**. It would be puzzling (though it is not completely out of the question) if he were to make a sudden detour to mention, in passing, his existential state of mind. Unfortunately, he does not complete the latter part of the sentence **'because I didn't have the...'** However, several possibilities do suggest themselves: 'because I didn't have the courage to be honest with people'; 'because I didn't have the resolve to confront the diagnosis'; 'because I didn't have the time/energy to fulfil my commitments'. If any of these (plausible) continuations was what Jack had in mind, if only vaguely, then 'I felt quite worthless' is an overstated version of 'I felt quite bad about myself', or perhaps 'I felt quite guilty'. It is clear that Jack, like most people, sometimes resorts to the clichés: 'paranoid' and 'shell-shocked' are two examples. It is not unlikely that this is another one.

The temptation to attribute special significance to *worthless* should be avoided. Rather than following SFL's tendency to latch on to the ideas of self and loss, and construing *worthless* as a reference to a loss of self-esteem, read what Jack says on either side of this sentence: **'I just felt that I couldn't, I felt like I'd lost something, I couldn't um, I just found everything so tiring, I couldn't.'** This is basically inarticulate groping. There is no consistent line of thought, and no sense of a core insight, or even a core experience, that Jack is trying to convey. However, there is a constant thread in one respect, and that is the sense of being disabled, which appears repeatedly in this speech: **I couldn't, I didn't have, I'd lost, I couldn't, I couldn't, I didn't have.** If there is a theme here, it seems to be that of lacking the resources – physical, cognitive, emotional – to deal with the diagnosis and its social consequences. It has nothing to do with the social construction of Jack's 'self'.

I felt like I'd lost something

This is just another of these half-thoughts, another fragment sandwiched between Jack's hesitant stumblings: I just felt that I couldn't ... I didn't have the ... I couldn't ... I just found everything so tiring

I couldn't um...

This phrase can be taken as another fragmented expression of the disability theme. Or it might be run together with the previous phrase: 'I felt like I'd lost something I couldn't um...', as if the thought was: 'I felt like I'd lost something I couldn't identify', or 'I felt like I'd lost something I could never get back'. Either way, the thought quickly peters out – as does every other thought in the first two speeches, with the exception of pretence/exhaustion. It is this latter idea to which Jack now reverts.

I just found everything so tiring, I couldn't, I didn't have anything to give,

He felt everything was tiring
Impact of diagnosis Something is happening which is almost catastrophic, the effects of diagnosis are very broad and much more than medical.

As I suggested earlier, this appears to continue what is arguably the prominent theme: being exhausted, feeling tired, having no energy, lacking resources, being disabled. Given what else he says, this tiredness is plausibly construed as the result of pretending to his friends that nothing was wrong, and trying not to think about his diagnosis. It is likely, of course, that symptoms arising from his physical condition will also have contributed to this loss of physical and mental energy. On this occasion, I have no problem with the SFL comments, except to query 'catastrophic'. No doubt Jack's diagnosis *was* a catastrophe. But I cannot see any reference to this in what he is saying here.

I didn't feel that I had anything worthwhile to kind of contribute or you know, the, I don't know,

Nothing was worthwhile
It seems strange to think of himself in a relational social way, this isn't about health but about what other people think of him? Deep impact of loss, grief, worth. In the past did he give a lot? What contribution is he talking about?

The descriptive comment added by SFL is interesting. They gloss this statement as meaning: 'Nothing was worthwhile'. But that is *not* what Jack appears to be saying. Feeling that you do not have anything worthwhile to contribute (to a project, for example) does *not* entail that you feel 'nothing is worthwhile'. So SFL are giving this observation a spin it doesn't have, in line with their constant search for anything that might signify a concern with existential themes: the self, identity, worthlessness, loss, and so on. A more plausible reading is that Jack is making a further reference to his 'lack of energy': everything is tiring, he feels exhausted, and he has nothing to give, nothing to contribute. It is variation on: 'I didn't, I hadn't, I couldn't...'

I was just kind of like shell-shocked I supposed, you know.

'Shell shock', first world war, horror, shock. Tremendous sense of difficulty. Impact of diagnosis.

This comment rounds off the second speech by using a familiar metaphor. Jack's diagnosis was akin to a detonation in his life; and the use of this metaphor suggests that the constant repetition of references to being disabled – I couldn't, I'd lost, I didn't have, I couldn't, I couldn't, I didn't have – may be the result of shock. This explanation is not identical to the other explanation he appears to offer (his lack of energy was caused by pretending that nothing was wrong, and trying not to think about the diagnosis), but it is certainly not incompatible with it. I do not think the 'shell-shocked' metaphor is particularly interesting, though SFL want to make something of it. It is a familiar cliché, used routinely to describe unpleasant surprises. In this case, it does refer to traumatic circumstances. However, in all probability Jack, like most people, has used it to characterise more mundane situations as well.

[sorry] So ... I don't know if that's answered the...

Tails off

The tailing off here is typical of Jack's hesitation, and his pattern of groping around for a suitable topic or continuation. Interestingly, he does not even finish the sentence: 'I don't know if that's answered the question'; and it's tempting to believe that this is another sign of his inability to work out precisely what is expected of him. Since the interviewer has given no indication of this, and (so far) no feedback either, his confusion and uncertainty are entirely understandable.

Third speech

Between the second speech and the third, the interviewer says something that is quite unlike what s/he has said earlier in the extract. It is different for three reasons. First, the interviewer checks that Jack is able to continue (this is what 'Are you up...?' seems to signify), and that he recognises 'the kind of style of questions that?' The latter is ironic, because it is certainly not clear from this extract what 'the style of questions' is supposed to be. So the fact that Jack replies in the affirmative ['yeah yeah'] may not indicate that he understands the 'style of question', but rather that he is 'up'. In other words, he is answering the 'Are you up...?' question, and is effectively giving the interviewer permission to continue.

Second, the interviewer very clearly signals approval of a certain fragment of what Jack has been saying. This is not the 'tiredness' narrative, which dominates Jack's replies so far, but (as the interviewer puts it) 'the sense of loss, a sense of being worthless or nothing being worthwhile'. Recall, however, that Jack never at any point suggested that 'nothing is worthwhile'. What he actually said is that he **'felt that he didn't have anything worthwhile to contribute'**, which is an expression of the 'tiredness' narrative. The 'Nothing was worthwhile' comment, added earlier in the transcript, is now reflected in the way that the interviewer changes Jack's own words into something more congenial to the IPA framework.

The approval is conveyed by 'you said some amazing things about...' In fact, this is rather more than just approval. It expresses praise, and is a mild form of flattery. It would require a kind of social blindness on Jack's part not to recognise this, if only subconsciously, and to respond to it by giving the interviewer more of the same. The interviewer's statement announces: 'That's what I want to hear about. Much more of that please.' Further observations on *loss, worthlessness* and *nothing being worthwhile* will obviously attract additional rewards.

Third, after another check that Jack is able to continue – 'are you alright with talking' [**'yeah yeah'**] – the interviewer finally asks an intelligible, specific and clear question: 'but what would you say that you had lost?' This question picks up Jack's statement, **'I felt that I'd lost something'**. As indicated above, this statement occurs in a series of hesitant fragments, stumbling half-thoughts never completed, as Jack tries to find a coherent line of thought that the interviewer will welcome. It is part of the **'I couldn't, I didn't, I'd lost, I didn't have'** thread. However, the interviewer has attached the 'what would you say that you had lost?' question to the *amazing things* comments; and this implies that Jack's answer to the question is most likely to be rewarded if it includes some reference to *worthlessness, nothing being worthwhile, loss*, and so on (or, more precisely, a reference to something that the interviewer can interpret in those terms).

> Ju just er ... what had I lost? Um...

> *Questions self, as if trying to get past the magnitude of his feelings and into the reality? Is he lost in thought and emotion of my questions?*

Jack's immediate response is more hesitation. It is not clear what thought might be lurking behind **Ju just er**. Just what? However, SFL appear to have no doubt. Their linguistic comment at this point says: 'Questions self, as if trying to get past the magnitude of his feelings'. It is just as plausible to suppose that Jack is not entirely sure what he meant by his earlier statement, **'I felt like I'd lost something'**, and is now trying to pin it down, asking himself exactly what it was he was referring to. **'What had I lost? Um.'** is further evidence for this interpretation. It is not unusual for people to say something and, when asked about it later, not be completely sure what they meant. So, in this case, Jack is casting around for a suitable response.

I'd lost the feeling that I had all the time in the world kind of, that I'd um ... I'd realised that at some point I was going to die, whether that was going to be 15, 20 how ever many years, I'd realised that that could happen and er ... I think that's what I'd lost.

A sense of emerging clarity in what had been lost. Language is clearer, easier and safer to say.
Impact of diagnosis Loss of future, <u>sense of mortality. Life expectation dramatically reduced idea of middle age and old age taken away? A new sense of the certainty of uncertainty in terms of mortality?</u>
<u>Clear awareness of much of the loss being in his own thinking about himself. His own beliefs about his worth. Deep implications of questioning his self.</u>

The first thought that strikes him is an aspect of the diagnosis he has not mentioned before (not in this extract, at least). It is the intimation of mortality, and the idea that his life expectancy has been reduced. His way of expressing this thought is compelling: 'I'd lost the feeling that I had all the time in the world'. This feeling is characteristic of the young; but, for Jack, the HIV diagnosis has taken it away. Instead of being able to think and act as if his death is an unimaginably long way into the future, he is now obliged to recognise that it will be at a determinate point – perhaps not imminent, but lurking over the horizon.

Typically, SFL embroider this: 'Clear awareness of the loss being in his own thinking about himself'. It would be difficult to argue that this sentence is inaccurate, but it does put a certain spin on Jack's words. The *loss* is the feeling of having all the time in the world; and although that is obviously something Jack thought about, it seems odd to say that the loss is 'in his own thinking about himself'. However, the rest of this comment – 'His own belief about his worth. Deep implications of questioning his self' – is purely imaginary, motivated by SFL's own theoretical commitments. There is nothing in Jack's response at this point that suggests a concern for his own 'worth', or that he is in any 'deep' sense questioning 'his self'. Here, as elsewhere, SFL import ideas rooted in their own theories, even if they claim to remain 'close to the text'.

Um ... but also I'd lost my self esteem and my self respect as well because, I'm not sure why um,

Lost self esteem Lost self respect
<u>Is he confused about what he went through and its cause?</u>

You can almost hear the change of gears in the first 'Um...' here. Jack's first response to the 'What would you say that you had lost?' question comes over as totally genuine. Apart from anything else, he devotes 57 words to it, the second longest passage on any single train of thought in the extract (after comments on 'whilst I was around ... really exhausting'). And 'I'd lost the feeling that I had all the time in the world' has a definiteness and originality that his other responses lack. At this point, however, there is a pause ... and his tentativeness returns. It is not hard to imagine him recalling (no doubt subconsciously) that what gets approval from the interviewer is something to do with the 'self' and 'worthlessness'. So he decides that he has lost his self esteem and self respect as well. Compared to the 'all the time in the world' observation, this is thin and unconvincing – as we might expect it to be, given that it is an attempt to win approval rather than an arresting and original form of self-expression. This is confirmed by how he continues: he'd lost his self-esteem and self-respect because ... well, because I'm not sure why um...

SFL take 'I'd lost my self esteem and my self respect as well' at face value, ignoring the social dynamics that have produced this response. 'Is he confused about what he went through and its cause?'... Well, almost certainly, yes. However, a great deal of Jack's confusion and uncertainty at this point reflects the fact that he is trying to please the interviewer without really knowing how to achieve this. He recognises, very broadly, what will win approval ('amazing things'); but his resources for self-understanding are not extensive enough for him to be able to produce the necessary material.

> Well because of the relationship that I was in but also because of the diagnosis definitely um ... it was a big big part of it.

Cause was partly his relationship (where he became infected) Cause was also diagnosis
Diagnosis major impact
Realizes multiple causes to this, the relationship and the diagnosis. Holistic and major impact of diagnosis.

Having admitted that he is not sure why he had lost his self esteem and my self respect, he now comes up with two possible explanations, although 'definitely um ... it was a big big part of it' sounds like an attempt to convince himself that the diagnosis genuinely explains, at least in part, his loss of self-esteem. In saying this, I am not arguing that Jack is mistaken in identifying the relationship and the diagnosis as causes of this loss. What I am arguing is that the way he talks about them is suggestive of a man who is admittedly not sure, and who is casting around for a plausible-sounding account. If, in general, it is true that people do not know the causes of their own psychological states, and that they often confabulate in order to 'fill in the gap', then Jack's response here seems to be a case in point.

Summary of the analysis

Much of what Jack says is stumbling, tentative, fragmented. Given my own background theories, I think this is a result of his uncertainty about what is wanted, and a lot of casting around to see what will please the interviewer (until he gets the 'amazing things' cue). SFL, meanwhile, regard it as a consequence of deep emotion, 'complexity', and a questioning of his 'self'. They say nothing about the dynamics of the interview, nor do they consider the extent to which Jack's responses are a function of the interview as a social process, rather than an indication of his 'inner' states.

SFL's attempt to find themes of identity, self, worthlessness and loss is constant, bordering on relentless. They employ a number of tactics in order to make it appear that these themes are derived from the data, instead of being 'imported' from non-interview sources.

For example, they try to work in 'self' at every opportunity, attaching it to 'paranoia', the reduction in life expectancy, any reference to thinking, any reference to 'loss', any reference to the diagnosis, any reference to other people ('Is the self social?'), and so on. When Jack suggests that he was paranoid about people knowing something was wrong, SFL translate this into a point about the self: '"Wrong", the old self was "right"?' They attach 'metaphysical' questions about the 'self' to every mundane thing Jack says. 'Who does the finding in finding themselves?'; 'Who are you if you're not yourself?'; 'Who is doing the performance?' Superficially, these questions appear to have a kind of 'existential depth'; but they are more akin to the questions you might find in adolescent attempts at poetry. On one occasion they misrepresent something Jack says. 'I didn't feel I had anything worthwhile to kind of contribute' is transformed into: 'Nothing was worthwhile'. On another occasion, they change the meaning of a verb Jack uses ('finding out' becomes 'finding') in order to be able to ask: 'If something was found what was lost?' In general, they either distort the data, or slant it in a way the text itself does not support. They are the research equivalent of spin doctors.

From my own perspective: in content analysis terms, Jack says most about: trying not to think about the diagnosis, pretending nothing was wrong, being exhausted, having nothing to contribute, and losing the feeling of having all the time in the world. There is a constant thread referring to the loss of resources: *I couldn't, I didn't have, I'd lost, I couldn't, I couldn't, I didn't, I didn't have*. The self-worthless-identity-loss cluster does not figure in this extract – except as a brief shot in the dark early on – until cued by the interviewer with 'amazing things'.

As I have said before, I am not arguing that the 'identity' interpretation is wrong (though I think it is), or that it is illegitimate to project it into the data. I am arguing that it cannot be derived from the data. It has to be imported, even though 'imported theory' is not something that SFL, officially, condone.

The absence of criteria

Conclusion: there is no *method* in IPA, any more than there is a method in Giorgi's modified Husserlian approach, or van Manen's hermeneutic phenomenology. In each case, the discourse of 'method' is a way of camouflaging a different kind of process; that is, finding in the text what you brought to it.

That's a rather blunt assessment, but let's take it bit by bit. First, there are some basic moves in each of the three approaches for which no specific instructions, and no specific criteria, are provided. Giorgi, for example, requires that as an initial step the data be divided into 'meaning units', representing the points at which the researcher 'experiences a shift of meaning'. He offers no criteria for identifying these shifts (and the discrepancies between the AG and BG versions suggest there aren't any). Van Manen suggests that the researcher should identify 'phrases that stand out', and sentences that 'seem to be thematic of the experience'. No criteria are given for what counts as 'standing out' or being 'thematic'. SFL propose that we should pick out key words and phrases, examine the 'semantic content', and 'note anything of interest'. They admit that 'there are no rules about what is commented on'. In all three cases, the initial step in the analysis – identifying meaning units, stand-out phrases, or things 'of interest' – is specified without *any* indication of how this can be done, or on what basis. It is left to each individual researcher to determine what counts as a shift in meaning, or something of interest, or a thematic sentence.

It is often suggested that this absence of criteria is a virtue. Qualitative research emphasises flexibility, openness, context, emergence, creativity, co-construction, and so on. However, the reality is that, where there are no specified criteria, rules, limits, or conditions, individuals will introduce their own. Into the vacuum created by the absence of logical criteria will rush a plethora of different assumptions, values, predilections and preferences, most of them unexamined, and all of them idiosyncratic to the researcher concerned. As a consequence, each analyst will find in the data a reflection of themselves.

Second, once 'meaning units', 'significant statements', or 'things of interest' have been picked out, the next step in all three approaches is a kind of semantic processing. In Giorgi's case, this is the 'meaning transformation'; for van Manen it is 'thematic formulation'; and for SFL it is 'conceptual annotating'.

The absence of criteria in the first phase is matched by a corresponding absence of criteria in the second. Giorgi says, explicitly, that he is not in the business of explaining how transformations are worked out. A transformation should express a 'heightened articulation of the psychological aspect of each meaning unit'; but we learn nothing about how this is achieved. According to van Manen, the researcher tries 'to unearth something "telling", something "meaningful", something "thematic"'; but he makes no attempt to explain how we can recognise what *is* 'meaningful', 'thematic' or 'telling'. Conceptual annotating, say SFL, will open up 'a range of provisional meanings'; but they do not explain how this 'opening up' is done. Nor do they say anything about how to distinguish between a 'provisional meaning' that fits the data and one that doesn't. They do suggest that 'it may be helpful to draw upon your own perceptions and understandings'. But they do not try to justify the claim that *this* person's 'perceptions' will help to elucidate *that* person's 'perceptions'. Or, put another way, the claim that *your* understandings are a guide to *someone else's* understandings.

In all three cases, we are informed we should identify, unearth, transform, or open up *meaning;* but we are given no coherent advice – we are given no advice at all – about how to do this.

But these decisions – picking out the key words or significant statements, doing conceptual annotation or meaning transformation – have to be made somehow, and on the basis of *some* criterion. If the writers of methodological texts do not, or cannot, specify criteria, then the researchers who perform the analysis will have to supply their own, whether consciously or unconsciously. If these researchers imagine that the 'meaning' they identify is 'based on a reading from within the text itself', then supplying their own criteria is more likely to be an unconscious process; and the meaning they find is likely to reflect their own agendas. For as Heidegger (1962: 150) observes:

> if when one is engaged in a particular kind of concrete interpretation ... one likes to appeal to what 'stands there', then one finds that what 'stands there' in the first instance is nothing other than the obvious undiscussed assumption of the person who does the interpreting.

So it is that, 'based on a reading from within the text itself', SFL discover the themes of identity and the 'self' everywhere they look, while van Manen finds confirmation of his beliefs about parenting. Giorgi is slightly different. He appears to have no obvious moral agenda (like van Manen), and no in-your-face theoretical commitments (like SFL). However, his apparent lack of emotional subtlety – for example, his inability to distinguish between different forms of jealousy, or between jealousy and envy, or between flirting and showing a romantic interest – restricts the range of 'meaning' he finds in his data.[4] For all of them, the absence of criteria makes their procedures arbitrary, and creates a vacuum into which personal idiosyncrasies can seep.

As a consequence of these idiosyncrasies, and the impetus to find favoured concepts 'standing there' (in Heidegger's terms), there is an inevitable tendency to misrepresent the data, whether by putting a greater semantic strain on the text than it will bear, or by ignoring the bits that don't fit, or by amplifying small fragments of the data, or by giving it a metaphysical spin, or by coaching the participant in the required responses, or sometimes by changing what the respondent said. Giorgi's conflation of jealousy and envy leads him to claim that the two emotions can be 'lived confusedly', and his wife to suggest that a person can be 'robbed' of something they 'already lack'. Van Manen seizes on a tangential reference to hope in a mother's story about how much pressure she should put on her son, and transforms it into a piece of devotional writing about pedagogy: 'Thus hope gives us pedagogy itself. Or is it pedagogy which grants us hope?' SFL change 'I didn't feel that I had anything worthwhile to kind of contribute' into 'nothing was worthwhile'. Considered superficially and in isolation, each of these could be depicted as a minor aberration; but, as I hope to have shown in this chapter and those on Giorgi and van Manen, this sort of data distortion is in fact endemic. It is a consequence of the absence of criteria, leading to a conceptual vacuum, leading to the unconscious intrusion of prior commitments and obsessions.

The conclusion that PQR's discourse of 'method' masks a different kind of process – that is, finding in the text what you brought to it – is not an unreasonable one. Antecedent theories are projected into the text, but the researcher is wedded to the assumption that a 'reading from within the text itself' produces concepts without any prompting from some 'external' theory. As a consequence, the true nature of the interpretive process remains concealed from both the reader and researcher. The latter imagines that she finds 'what's in the text'. The former defers to her authority.

Interpretation, making inferences about text, is only possible with the help of a background theory. The idea that it is an achievement of 'hermeneutics', close attention to the text, or an 'interpretive method', is a phenomenological myth.

Notes

1 There three other reasons. One is an unconscious deference to authorial authority. Another is that, in many published research reports, there is just not enough illustrative data, and not enough discussion of the creation of codes/categories, to be able to undertake a proper evaluation. The third is a reluctance to do the hard yards: to scrutinise thoroughly the researcher's data alongside her codes and categories. The kind of work I do in this chapter, and in the chapters on Giorgi and van Manen, is done rather rarely.
2 There is another, very instructive, example of this kind of thing in Packer (2011: 59–60), a discussion of an illustrative bit of coding in Auerbach and Silverstein (2003).
3 I don't mean to imply that I originated these theories, only that I am prepared to sign up to them. The title of this section is a reference to a well-known Monty Python sketch.
4 To be fair to Giorgi, he does try to carry out a 'reading from within the text' without invoking any 'external' theories. However, because that gives him nothing on which to base a 'meaning' inference, he is reduced to proposing arbitrary synonyms and minor adjustments in syntax. In an effort to comply with the axiom of resident meaning, he unwittingly shows that it cannot be complied with. The oddities of the 'structures' produced by Giorgi and his wife come from welding the two stories together, and from their failure to recognise the emotional nuances in both.

References

Antaki, C., and Rapley, M. (1996) ' "Quality of life" talk: the liberal paradox of psychological testing', *Discourse and Society*, 7(3), pp. 293–316.

Auerbach, C. F., and Silverstein, L. B. (2003) *Qualitative Data: An Introduction to Coding and Analysis*. New York: New York University Press.

Baker, C. (2001) 'Ethnomethodological analyses of interviews', in J. F. Gubrium, and J. A. Holstein (eds.) *Handbook of Interview Research: Context and Method*. London: Sage, pp. 777–796.

Buunk, A. P., and Van Vugt, M. (2013) *Applying Social Psychology: From Problems to Solutions*. 2nd edition. Los Angeles: Sage.

Carruthers, P. (2011) *The Opacity of Mind: An Integrative Theory of Self-Knowledge*. Oxford: Oxford University Press.

Doris, J. M. (2015) *Talking to Our Selves: Reflection, Ignorance, and Agency*. Oxford: Oxford University Press.

Edwards, D. (1997) *Discourse and Cognition*. London: Sage.

Feldman Barrett, L. (2006) 'Are emotions natural kinds?', *Perspectives on Psychological Science*, 1(1), pp. 28–58.

Flowers, P., Davis, M., Hart, G., Rosengarten, M., Frankis, J., and Imrie, J. (2006) 'Diagnosis and stigma and identity amongst HIV positive Black Africans living in the UK', *Psychology & Health*, 21(1), pp. 109–122.

Glaser, B. G., and Strauss, A. L. (1967) *The Discovery of Grounded Theory: Strategies for Qualitative research.* New Brunswick: Aldine Transaction.

Grice, P. (1991) *Studies in the Way of Words.* Cambridge, MA: Harvard University Press.

Hassin, R. R., Uleman, J. S., and Bargh, J. A. (eds.) (2005) *The New Unconscious.* New York: Oxford University Press.

Heidegger, M. (1962) *Being and Time.* Oxford: Basil Blackwell.

Holloway, I., and Wheeler, S. (2010) *Qualitative Research in Nursing and Healthcare.* 3rd edition. Oxford: Wiley-Blackwell.

Kahneman, D. (2011) *Thinking, Fast and Slow.* London: Allen Lane.

Krippendorff, K.H. (2013) *Content Analysis: An Introduction to its Methodology.* Thousand Oaks, CA: Sage.

Kunda, Z. (1999) *Social Cognition: Making Sense of People.* Cambridge, MA: MIT Press.

Kvale, S., and Brinkman, S. (2009) *InterViews: Learning the Craft of Qualitative Research Interviewing.* 2nd edition. Los Angeles: Sage.

Larkin, M., and Griffiths, M. D. (2002) 'Experiences of addiction and recovery: the case for subjective accounts', *Addiction Research and Theory*, 10(3), pp. 281–311.

Mead, G. H. (1934) *Mind, Self, and Society from the Standpoint of a Social behaviorist.* Chicago: University of Chicago Press.

Mills, C. W. (1940) 'Situated actions and vocabularies of motive', *American Sociological Review*, 5(6), pp. 904–913.

Myers, G. (2004) *Matters of Opinion: Talking About Public Ideas.* Cambridge, UK: Cambridge University Press.

Nisbett, R. E., and Wilson, T. D. (1977) 'Telling more than we can know: verbal reports on mental processes', *Psychological Review*, 84(3), pp. 231–259.

Packer, M. (2011) *The Science of Qualitative Research.* Cambridge, UK: Cambridge University Press.

Potter, J., and Hepburn, A. (2005) 'Qualitative interviews in psychology: problems and possibilities', *Qualitative Research in Psychology*, 2(4), pp. 281–307.

Rapley, T. J. (2001) 'The art(fulness) of open-ended interviewing: some considerations on analysing interviews', *Qualitative Research*, 1(3), pp. 303–323.

Riffe, D., Lacy, S., and Fico, F. (2013) *Analyzing Media Messages: Using Quantitative Content Analysis in Research.* 3rd edition. New York: Routledge.

Sabini, J., Siepmann, M., and Stein, J. (2001) 'The really fundamental attribution error in social psychological research', *Psychological Inquiry*, 12(1), pp. 1–15.

Schwitzgebel, E. (2011) *Perplexities of Consciousness.* Cambridge, MA: MIT Press.

Sinclair, J. M. (1997) 'Corpus evidence in language description', in A. Wichmann, S. Fligelstone, T. McEnery, and G. Knowles (eds.) *Teaching and Language Corpora.* London: Longman, pp. 27–39.

Smith, J. A. (1994) 'Reconstructing selves: an analysis of discrepancies between women's contemporaneous and retrospective accounts of the transition to motherhood', *British Journal of Psychology*, 85(3), pp. 371–392.

Smith, J. A. (1999) 'Identity development during the transition to motherhood: An interpretative phenomenological analysis', *Journal of Reproductive and Infant Psychology*, 17(3), pp. 281–289.

Smith, J.A., Flowers, P., and Larkin, M. (2009) *Interpretative Phenomenological Analysis.* London: Sage.

Smith, J.A., and Osborn, M. (2007) 'Pain as an assault on the self: An interpretative phenomenological analysis of the psychological impact of chronic benign low back pain', *Psychology & Health*, 22(5), pp. 517–535.

Sperber, D., and Wilson, D. (1995) *Relevance: Communication and Cognition.* Oxford: Blackwell.

Teddlie, C., and Tashakkori, A. (2009) *Foundations of Mixed Methods Research: Integrating Quantitative and Qualitative Approaches in the Social and Behavioural Sciences.* Los Angeles: Sage.

van den Berg, H., Wetherell, M., and Houtkoop-Steenstra, H. (eds.) (2003) *Analyzing Race Talk: Multidisciplinary Approaches to the Interview.* Cambridge, UK: Cambridge University Press.

Vazire, S., and Wilson, T. D. (eds.) (2012) *Handbook of Self-Knowledge.* New York: The Guilford Press.

Weber, R. P. (1990) *Basic Content Analysis.* 2nd edition. Newbury Park, CA: Sage.

Widdowson, H. G. (2004) *Text, Context, Pretext: Critical Issues in Discourse Analysis.* Oxford: Blackwell Publishing.

Wierzbicka, A. (2006) *English: Meaning and Culture.* Oxford: Oxford University Press.

Wilson, T. D. (2002) *Strangers to Ourselves: Discovering the Adaptive Unconscious.* Cambridge, MA: The Belknap Press of Harvard University Press.

Zawidzki, T. W. (2013) *Mindshaping: A New Framework for Understanding Human Social Cognition.* Cambridge, MA: The MIT Press,.

7   Meaning, models and mechanisms

Once we have a clear understanding of what meaning is – or, rather, once we understand the linguistic function of the words 'means' and 'meaning' – the phenomenological picture described in Chapter 2 quickly unravels. In particular, the axiom of resident meaning must be abandoned. The idea that 'there is an underlying meaning inherent in the text itself which is not directly accessible to readers, but which exegetic authority can reveal' (Widdowson 2004: 129) has to go.[1] The reason why 'resident meaning' is 'hidden' in the text has now become clear. It was never resident in the first place. It was brought in from outside.

This is confirmed by an examination of the three methodological texts I have considered. All of them fail to comply with the axiom of resident meaning, even though they explicitly endorse it. Giorgi is the author who makes the biggest effort to *not* go beyond the text, and to 'understand the meaning of the description based solely on what is present in the data'. But, lacking the resource of a theory on which to base 'meaning attribution' inferences, he is reduced to arbitrary synonyms and trivial adjustments to syntax. Unlike the other authors, he genuinely stays within the text; but, for that very reason, he can find no significant 'meaning'. Changing 'in the lunch group that he went out with' to 'with whom he went out to lunch' is about the best he can do; and his claim that the second of these expressions conveys the 'psychological aspect' of the experience in a 'heightened articulation' stretches credulity to the limits.

Giorgi sticks to the text, but engenders no meaning. In contrast, van Manen and SFL engender meaning, but only by going beyond the text. SFL have unacknowledged recourse to a theory of identity derived from the work of Mead, according to which a self 'comes into being through social interaction with others', and which implies that 'no hard-and-fast line can be drawn between our own selves and the selves of others'. They look for confirmation of this theory in every line of the HIV interview, warping the text where necessary in order to accommodate it. Meanwhile, van Manen brings his own theories about parenting to the data. In the 'being left, being abandoned' example, he places 'dropping your child off at school' and 'abandoning them permanently' (as in *Sophie's Choice* or *Hansel and Gretel*) in the same category; and in his analysis of Robert's mother's narrative, he takes a tangential reference to 'hope', and turns it into a lengthy, quasi-Pauline epistle. In both cases, meaning is certainly propagated; but only by ditching the axiom of resident meaning, and implicitly appealing to external theories.[2]

The appeal to theory is not confined to meaning attribution in this primary sense. As was evident in the 'Diane and Keith' example in Chapter 6, theory determines the categories according to which items of data are classified. In identifying 'units of information with similar content', a theory of some kind must be invoked to delimit what will count as relevantly 'similar'. This delimitation does not just emerge from the data itself, despite the expression 'emergent themes'. Data/text does not somehow incorporate the relevant criteria-for-similarity which can be used to analyse it. Such criteria are no more resident in the data/text than meaning is. They have to be specified from some external perspective.[3]

I take it, then, that recourse to an external theory – 'external' in the sense that it is not intrinsic to, and cannot be derived from, the data – is inevitable in qualitative analysis. From this point of view, the most familiar way of understanding the contrast between 'deductive' and 'inductive' forms of social research does not stand up. If 'inductive' means that 'theory is the *outcome* of research' (Bryman 2016: 22), and if the implication of this is that *no* antecedent theory can be used in an inductive study, then research can never be purely inductive.[4]

What is a phenomenon?

However, as earlier chapters have suggested, it is not just in the analysis phase of a research study that meaning attribution occurs. It is also implicated in the initial specification of a phenomenon-for-study. The identification of a phenomenon *itself* presupposes an antecedent theory, held by the researcher or by a community of researchers. Meaning attribution, the inference that the researcher makes on the basis of the antecedent theory, is the basis for how the 'phenomenon' is defined in the first place.

The most dramatic example of this was discussed in Chapter 4. Van Manen identifies a phenomenon that he refers to as the child's experience of 'feeling left or abandoned'. He selects several instances of this phenomenon to serve as the data/text for a thematic formulation (which ultimately turns out to be 'homelessness, brokenness'). However, the question is: on what basis does he suppose that 'feeling left or abandoned' *is* a 'phenomenon'? The instances of it that he presents range from dropping a child off at school to abandoning a child permanently, as in *Hansel and Gretel*, or *Housekeeping* (the Marilynne Robinson novel, in which a lone parent, the mother, commits suicide). How does van Manen justify placing such different situations *in the same category*? Well, as I suggested at the time, he doesn't. He just lumps them all together and, without bothering to explain his reasoning, says: these are examples of the 'same phenomenon'.

In presenting these cases as instances of the same phenomenon, van Manen is already giving notice of what his analysis will be. The underlying message is: dropping off your children at school, or at the day centre, is like abandoning them permanently. It is akin to committing suicide, or absenting yourself for ever after a divorce. It has that kind of significance for the child – and for the parent. The definition of the phenomenon carries an emotionally loaded message: 'Every time you leave a child with a babysitter, or at the day care centre, you are doing something that is comparable to abandoning them permanently, just as the daughter in *Sophie's Choice* was abandoned'. Van Manen's views on parenting are already implicit in the examples of the 'phenomenon' he has chosen.

This, as I have observed, is a dramatic example; but the point I am making can be generalised. When we identify anything as 'a phenomenon', we are doing so on the basis of some theory. Not just *any* form of words picks out a phenomenon. 'Accidentally breaking pencils and putting two rhinoceroses in a bag' is a coherent form of words, but it does not specify a 'phenomenon'. It is not, as the philosophers say, a natural kind.[5] To identify a phenomenon for study, there must be some antecedent theory that justifies placing a certain group of items in the same category.

The relevant theory will almost always be a causal one:

> [P]icking out a phenomenon has something to do with distinguishing the causal processes that make up that phenomenon ... if we observe rain falling, asking what causes the rain is the first step of turning this observation into something that constitutes a phenomenon.
>
> (Bailer-Jones 2009: 160)

So identifying the phenomenon involves a type of inference. Instances of the phenomenon belong in the same category because there is reason to believe that they participate in similar causal processes.

This means that, in both the natural and social sciences, the antecedent theory is often based on earlier studies. As Bailer-Jones points out: 'that something is identified as a phenomenon is, in many instances, already the result of research' (162). It is only possible to take an interest in the melting point of lead (327° C) as a phenomenon, and ask why lead melts at that particular temperature, because studies have been conducted in which 327° C is a consistent and reliable finding (Haynes 2015). Similarly, we can only refer to the phenomenon of declining church attendance in the UK because previous studies have already identified and measured this decline (Bruce 2013, Franck and Iannaccone 2014).

Many PQR studies, probably most, do not succeed in identifying a phenomenon in this sense. At best, they identify a *topic*, not a phenomenon. Consider some 'phenomena' studied in recent PQR research:

Recovery from breast cancer-related breast surgery (Elmir *et al.* 2010)

Caring in formal care for women with alcohol dependency (Thurang *et al.* 2010)

Being taken care of by nurses and physicians for relatives in Norwegian intensive care units (Frivold *et al.* 2015)

Empowerment of nursing students in clinical practice (Bradbury-Jones *et al.* 2010)

Family communication of *BRCA1/2* results (Crotser and Dickerson 2010)

The transition process of new nurses in Taiwan (Lee *et al.* 2013)

The experience of registered psychiatric nurses in the province of Manitoba, Canada (Jackson and Morrissette 2014)

Professional competence experienced by Norwegian nurse students (Thorkildsen and Råholm 2010)

None of these 'phenomena' makes even an implicit reference to a set of research findings. Unlike 'the melting point of lead' or 'the decline of church attendance in the UK', they are not associated with any specific claim for which there is evidence. 'The melting point of lead' is associated with the claim that lead melts at 327° C. 'The decline of church attendance in the UK' is associated with the claim that (for example) between 40 and 60 per cent of the adult population attended church regularly in 1851, whereas only 7.5 per cent did so in 1998.[6] But what are the corresponding claims for 'empowerment of nursing students in clinical practice', and 'professional competence experienced by Norwegian nurse students'?

Inevitably, the authors of such studies talk about 'exploring' the topic, or 'gaining insight' into it, or 'acquiring further understanding'. This is their research aim. In contrast, 'the melting point of lead' suggests a very specific question: Why does lead melt at 327° C? 'The decline of church attendance in the UK' suggests another one: What accounts for this decline? None of the topics listed above suggests a specific question in this way. So the authors resort to the vaguest of gestures: 'to develop new insights into the phenomenon' (Atsalos *et al.* 2014). Ask the respondents to talk about the designated topic, and hope that they come up with something that can be represented as interesting.

Theories, data, models

I am making a case for the claim that theory, in some form, is unavoidable in qualitative research.

First, a phenomenon cannot be specified in the absence of a theory or findings from previous research. Topics can be alluded to, and how they are defined may well rest on views that the researcher already holds – as in the case of van Manen. But a topic is not a phenomenon. To specify a phenomenon, reference must be made to a plausible theory and/or well established findings.

Second, data analysis cannot be carried out without some theoretical perspective (in Heidegger's terms, this is *Vorsicht*). Analytical categories do not 'emerge' without theoretical prompting. The data does not somehow contain instructions for how the data can be analysed; nor can the relevant categories simply be read off from the text.

Third, any attempt to elucidate the 'meaning of the phenomenon' must draw on a theory. Meaning is not resident in the data; the text's 'deeper narrative' cannot be distilled, illuminated, unearthed, uncovered, or unconcealed by an expert in hermeneutics.

The alternative approach I will present in the remainder of this chapter will explicitly acknowledge the significance of theory in qualitative research. However, there is a slight difficulty to be overcome before I start. This arises from the fact that discussions of theory in the context of qualitative methods are often bedevilled by what looks like an outmoded view of 'deduction' and 'induction'.

A distinction is typically drawn between a 'top-down' approach and a 'bottom-up' approach. According to this view, 'top' and 'up' refer to theory, while 'down' and 'bottom' refer to data. The idea is that the researcher either starts with a theory, and then generates data ('top-down'), or starts with data, and then generates a theory to account for it ('bottom-up').

For example, Bryman (2016: 23) suggests that *deduction* entails a ('top-down') process in which

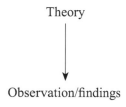

By contrast, in *induction*, 'the connection is reversed' (bottom-up):

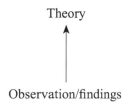

The idea is that the researcher 'deduces' a hypothesis from the theory, and then the research is designed to test that hypothesis. The findings may either confirm or disconfirm the hypothesis (and, in the latter case, might imply that the theory needs to be modified). This is called 'deductive research', or 'deduction', or the 'hypothetico-deductive method'. In contrast, the bottom-up approach, which is more characteristic of qualitative studies, 'starts with empirical particulars on the ground, and generates more general theories at a higher level' (Moses and Knutsen 2012: 22). This approach is called 'induction', or 'inductive research', or sometimes 'theory-generating'/'theory-building' research.

I said that this view looks outmoded because it originates with positivist accounts of scientific method, and ignores recent work on models in philosophy of science (examples include: Mayo 1996; Morgan and Morrison 1999; Giere 2006; Hartmann *et al.* 2008; Bailer-Jones 2009; and Weisberg 2013). Whether we opt for deduction ('top-down') or induction ('bottom-up'), the implication is that a theory is the main point of reference for what we know about the world. As Bailer-Jones (2008: 17) observes: 'Tradition has it that theories are carriers of knowledge telling us what the empirical world is like'. The function of data is to provide evidential support for a theory, call it T, either by testing a hypothesis derived from T, or by serving as the raw material out of which T is constructed. Either way, T is what we are aiming at. The data set is important mainly because it provides evidence for or against the theory.

This positivist account has been superseded, thanks mainly to a closer observation of scientific practice. Theories are too general, and often too abstract, to serve as 'knowledge carriers', at least in the context of specific bits of the world. Rather, it is models that do the real work, mediating between the theory, in all its abstraction, and the particular-concrete segment of the world that interests us. The usual day-to-day business of scientific enquiry – what Kuhn called 'normal science' – is to show how a given theory fits a certain chunk of the world by devising a model.

Although it is not the only purpose models have, this function – to show how a theory can be applied to a particular phenomenon – is one of the most important.

Fisher's Principle, for example, is an evolutionary model of sex ratios among species that produce offspring through sexual reproduction. It explains the following phenomenon: 'Among such species the sex ratio is approximately $1:1$'. This is Hamilton's (1967: 477) classic account of it:

1   Suppose male births are less common than female.
2   A newborn male then has better mating prospects than a newborn female, and therefore can expect to have more offspring.
3   Therefore parents genetically disposed to produce males tend to have more than average numbers of grandchildren born to them.
4   Therefore the genes for male-producing tendencies spread and male births become commoner.
5   As the $1:1$ sex ratio is approached, the advantage associated with producing males dies away.
6   The same reasoning holds if females are substituted for males throughout. Therefore $1:1$ is the equilibrium ratio.

Like all models, the Fisher Principle only works when certain conditions are met (for example, there must be population-wide competition for mates). However, it illustrates the way in which Darwinian natural selection can be applied to the specific phenomenon of 1 : 1 sex ratios in sexually reproducing species.

In more general terms, it also illustrates the way in which models are devised by assembling 'some bits of theories, some bits of empirical evidence', perhaps a bit of mathematical formalism, and a metaphor. (Morrison and Morgan 1999: 13). As Frigg and Hartmann (2012) suggest: models 'are neither derived entirely from data nor from theory. Model building is an art not a mechanical procedure.'

As the extract from Morrison and Morgan implies, the construction of a model very often involves more than one theory and possibly several sources of data. This is another important difference between the model-centred view of science and the 'top-down' and 'bottom-up' accounts. We can picture it as in Figure 7.1.

Mechanisms

Some models, as in the sex-ratio example, incorporate one or more *mechanisms* suggested by a relevant theory.[7] The idea that the special sciences – especially biology, but also psychology and sociology – search for mechanisms rather than universal laws has been widely discussed in recent philosophy of science (Craver and Darden 2013; Bechtel and Richardson 2010) and social theory (Hedström and Swedberg 1998; Elster 2007).

A mechanism is a process that reliably brings about a change from one state to another state. Identifying a mechanism explains a phenomenon by 'showing the cogs and wheels of the internal machinery' (Elster 1983: 24–5), indicating how event A leads to event B, which leads to event C … and so on. This is obviously a metaphorical description, and the main conceptual reference point is machines with contiguous moving parts. For example, the movement of a bicycle can be explained by showing how pressure on the pedals moves the crank arms, which rotate the crankset, which rotates the drive chain, which

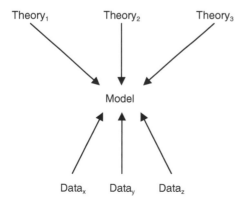

Figure 7.1 Theories, data and models.

(through its connection to the cogset) rotates the rear wheel. By metaphorical extension, however, the idea of a mechanism can be applied to biological, psychological and social phenomena.

Consider one type of psychological mechanism. In certain circumstances, people can be subject to a particular form of psychological discomfort. These circumstances generally involve an inconsistency between two different 'cognitions' the individual has, a particularly interesting case being where one of the cognitions concerns the individual's behaviour. For example, a belief the individual has, or a value that she holds dear, is inconsistent with something she has actually done. The discomfort generated by the inconsistency is such that the person concerned is strongly motivated to reduce it. This state of discomfort is known as 'cognitive dissonance' (Cooper 2007; Gawronski 2012).

The individual concerned can reduce the dissonance in one of several ways. The main options are:

1   Change your behaviour
2   Change your belief
3   Rationalise your behaviour by referring to a particular aspect of the environment

The vast majority of psychological studies of cognitive dissonance focus on option [2]. This is perhaps the most interesting and unexpected choice; but it turns out that, in many situations, changing your belief is the preferred (if unconscious) strategy for reducing dissonance. Indeed, 'cognitive dissonance' is sometimes used to refer to option [2], rather than to the state of discomfort it is intended to relieve.

Suppose, for example, that I am participating in an experimental study, and that I have just told another experimental subject that the task they are about to perform is fun. This is inconsistent with the fact that I have already rated it as tedious. It is not possible to change my behaviour [option 1] because this is a one-off. However, imagine that the experimenter paid me $150 to mislead the other subject in this way. In that case, I can explain my behaviour – and thereby reduce the dissonance – by citing a significant financial incentive [option 3]. Now, though, imagine that the experimenter paid me only $5. That is not a strong enough incentive to account for my behaviour, so option [3] is ruled out. The only option I am left with is to reduce the dissonance by amending, or reversing, my belief about the task [option 2]. So when I'm asked to rate the task again, I score it as interesting. This is an abbreviated account of a classic experiment by Festinger and Carlsmith (1959). Subjects who were paid $150 to mislead the other subject did not subsequently change their evaluation of the task. Subjects who were paid only $5 did.[8]

So cognitive dissonance functions as a mechanism. The cognitive inconsistency produces psychological discomfort, which the individual concerned is strongly motivated to eliminate or reduce. As a result, in certain circumstances, she unconsciously changes her beliefs.[9] This does not happen on every occasion;

but the situations in which it does happen can be studied. There are no ropes and pulleys here, no chains and cogwheels; but the idea of one event recognisably leading to another is the same.

Before closing this section, I will draw attention to a useful distinction made by Craver (2007), who contrasts what he calls *how-possibly* models with *how-actually* models. 'How-possibly' models are 'loosely constrained conjectures' about what sort of mechanism might be capable of producing the phenomenon (112). 'How-actually' models are supported by better evidence, and 'describe real components, activities, and organisational features' of the mechanism. In the approach to qualitative research outlined in the rest of this chapter, 'how-possibly' models play a significant part.

To summarise the discussion of this section. If, as I have suggested, theory is an inevitable component of qualitative research, its function will not correspond to the 'top-down'/'bottom-up' framework of 'deduction versus induction'. Instead, theories of various kinds will be implicated in models that the researcher formulates, particularly models depicting 'how-possibly' mechanisms. If we are to abandon the axiom of resident meaning, this is the direction in which I think we should proceed.

In the remainder of this chapter, I present an extended example of my own, based on a published PQR paper (Tavakol *et al.* 2012). The idea is to briefly review how this study was carried out, and with what result, and then develop an alternative approach. I have chosen this paper for three reasons. First, it is relatively straightforward, and will not involve a lot of tangential complexities. Second, it is in two or three key respects typical of the PQR literature. Third, it has a topical and important theme: empathy in health care.

The next section summarises the paper, and adds a few comments in italics.

Medical students' understanding of empathy: a phenomenological study

The study begins with the observation that there is no consensus about the meaning of empathy in the medical education literature, although it is generally agreed that empathy is conducive to positive health care outcomes. However, the authors suggest, one could argue that empathy is not compatible with the Oslerian paradigm of 'detached concern'.

Most empirical studies of empathy have used quantitative methods and self-report instruments. These methods do not permit in-depth inquiry, or provide an opportunity to explore the views and attitudes of medical staff and students. 'The nature of an individual's social reality ... cannot be understood from statistical procedures', and empathy is a psychosocial phenomenon that 'should be investigated in a natural setting in order to capture the complexities of human experience' (Tavakol *et al.* 2012: 307).

This is a typical example of qualitative research discourse. In practice, the study adopts a frequency-distribution approach (see Chapter 2), reducing '373 significant meaning units' to a smaller number of categories. In broad terms, this is a statistical procedure. Interviews were conducted in private rooms at a medical education unit. It isn't clear why this counts as a natural setting in which complex human experiences can be captured.

So the authors conducted a 'phenomenological study of the empathy experiences of undergraduates'. An important factor in selecting this population is that previous research reported a decline in mean empathy scores at the end of Year 3. A total of ten volunteer medical students, recruited by a message posted in the school's virtual learning environment, were interviewed, although 'we recruited medical students until we attained information redundancy or saturation.' Seven students were in Year 4, three were in Year 5. They were asked: 'Can you tell me how you see empathy in the context of patient care?' 'Can you tell me how you deal with the emotional state of the patient?' 'Can you tell me how empathy can be enhanced during medical education?'

I have commented on saturation in Chapter 2, note 16. The last of the three questions is unexpected. How would medical students assess methods of enhancing empathy? Would they refer to experimental evidence, for example? Would they even be aware of such evidence? Or would they just offer their own opinions? If the latter, what would those opinions be based on?

The analysis of transcripts 'was grounded in the procedures developed by Colaizzi and Giorgi'. The authors identified 'units of meaning' that 'exemplified students' essential meanings and experiences of empathy', and 'extracted a total of 373 significant meaning units'

The authors do not explain how this was done, or provide criteria for determining 'essential meanings' and 'significant meaning units'.

The findings were presented as five central themes, which I will label from (a) to (e).

(a) Participants interpreted the concept of empathy in different ways.

(b) Participants 'showed positive attitudes towards the importance of demonstrating empathy in the context of patient care'.

If (a) is true, it is not clear what significance (b) has. Some participants might be positive towards one understanding of 'empathy'; others might be positive towards a quite different understanding. It is clear, reading excerpts from the transcripts, that the students are not all talking about the same thing, even though they use the same word. Given that there is no consensus about the 'meaning of empathy' in the literature, it is not surprising that students produce disparate accounts as well.

(c) Most of the participants stated 'that the capacity for empathy arises from a natural attribute, and is governed by a person's temperament and upbringing'. But a few participants described 'the importance of education for enhancing natural empathy'. The authors suggest that 'these comments draw attention to the fact that students have insight into the qualities that make a good empathiser'.

What do the students mean by a 'natural attribute', and how do they know that empathy is one? If they have not read the relevant studies – they are not reported as citing any – we might conclude that they are just expressing their own opinions. In which case, what are these opinions based on? It is not clear why the authors think that the students 'have insight into the qualities that make a good empathiser', particularly as (a) implies that they don't all understand 'empathy' in the same way.

(d) Students 'had different experiences of and explanations for the decline or enhancement of empathy' during medical education.

Again, this is hardly surprising if they interpret 'empathy' in different ways, as theme (a) suggests. One student, interpreting 'empathy' as X, might report a decline. Another student, interpreting 'empathy' as Y, might report an enhancement. Is it self-evident that they have had 'different experiences' of the same thing?

(e) Participants 'had difficulties with the methods and timing of some of the learning opportunities in the curriculum'. They preferred to 'improve their empathy skills by observing the role modelling of teachers and through clinical experiential learning'.

In fact, most of the transcript excerpts refer primarily to communication skills training. According to the authors' own discussion of what 'empathy' means (in their introduction), it is not clear that empathy can be construed as a 'communication skill' (though it may improve communication skills).

In the discussion section, the authors say that the aim of the study was to 'explore the essence of [the students'] understanding of empathy'. The students, they suggest, 'believe empathy to be a combination of understanding, experience and imagination that helps an individual deal with the internal feelings and emotions of a patient'. It is an innate capacity that can be enhanced by learning. However, the authors also point out that 'some participants did not distinguish between empathy and sympathy'.

Earlier, the authors say that 'the final themes were then synthesised to elucidate the essential structure of the phenomenon of empathy'. There is a slide here from 'the essence of empathy' to 'the essence of the students' understanding of empathy'. However, it is not clear that the essence of X and the essence of someone's understanding of X are identical. The 'essence of the students' understanding' turns out to be a series of beliefs that the students expressed. However, if some of the students did not distinguish between sympathy and empathy, then some of them presumably believe that it is sympathy, not empathy, that is a 'combination of understanding, experience and imagination'. Throughout the paper, it must be the case that, when some of the participants refer to 'empathy', it is sympathy that they have in mind.

The conclusion suggests that, according to the findings, 'the ability to display empathy depends on the possession of innate empathic ability and the provision of empathy education for students'. So clinical teachers 'should value the importance of empathy', and the element of experiential learning 'should be considered by medical educators'. Students 'should be given the time and space to observe, acquire and demonstrate empathic skills'.

Note the generalisation ('the ability to display empathy depends...'), and the 'should' epidemic. Recall that these are based on the opinions of ten self-selected students from a single institution. Note also the slide from 'We capture lifeworld experiences rather than objective data' (307) to the assumption that it is legitimate to act ('clinical teachers should...') on the basis of what these ten students 'believe'. It is a slide from data about 'subjective perceptions' to recommendations about what should happen in the 'objective' world. As I suggested in Chapter 2, this is a general tendency in PQR studies (Paley 2005).

The remainder of this chapter is devoted to outlining an alternative study on the following phenomenon: the decline of empathy in medical students. I will take some clues from the Tavakol *et al.* paper, borrow a few bits of theory and data from social psychology, and try to construct a 'how-possibly' model that is capable of explaining an interesting phenomenon rather than simply exploring a topic.

However, my aim is not so much to get the model right as to trace the thought processes that lead to its construction.

The decline of empathy in medical students: the phenomenon

Empathy, or 'the essence of the students' understanding of empathy', is not a phenomenon but a topic. Without a specific question derived from previous research, Tavakol *et al.* (2012) have little choice but to talk about identifying the students' 'experiences of the phenomenon of empathy', and exploring 'the essence of their empathy'. This is a 'gaining further insight' study: invite a small sample of people to talk about their experiences of empathy, and hope – despite the fact that there is already vast literature on the topic – that something new turns up.

So the first thing to do is identify a *phenomenon*, something that implies a specific question that we can attempt to answer.

The question should be such that an answer to it would be useful. It would imply taking action *A* rather than action *B*, or adopting policy *F* rather than policy *G*. I don't think the answer to the question 'What is the essence of the students' understanding of empathy?' meets this requirement.[10] Nor does 'What is the essence of their empathy?' or 'What do medical students experience to be the essence or essential structure of empathy?' (These are all expressions that Tavakol *et al.* employ, even though 'the essence of empathy', 'the essence of the understanding of empathy', and 'the experience of the essence of empathy' don't look as if they refer to the same thing.)

It is my hypothesis, but not something I can demonstrate, that clues to an interesting phenomenon can nearly always be found in the introduction or background sections of any PQR paper. It is not that PQR authors are unaware of potentially relevant research; it is rather that they are obliged to ignore it because PQR ideology forces them down the path of 'exploring experiences of X' and/or 'exploring the essence of X'. Often, an author appears to be on the verge of pinpointing an interesting question, when all of a sudden she draws a line under the discussion, and jumps to: 'Therefore, a study of the experience of X was undertaken'. The interesting question with a potentially useful answer disappears, and the one-size-fits-all PQR research aim takes its place.

The Tavakol *et al.* paper is a case in point, because the interesting phenomenon begins to suggest itself on the first page. Two of the authors are faculty members in a university medical education unit, which provides them with a rather obvious perspective.[11] So it is not surprising that, following some opening remarks on 'the meaning of empathy in the medical education literature', they should refer to 'a 5-year longitudinal study of 456 medical students', which showed that mean empathy scores declined at the end of Year 3 (Hojat *et al.* 2009). Since the authors opted to interview students in Years 4 and 5, the obvious question is: Why not adopt a more *specific* research question? Something like: 'Why do mean empathy scores decline at the end of Year 3?' Why settle for what is, in contrast, a pointlessly general research objective: 'to investigate undergraduate medical students' experiences of the phenomenon of empathy during the course of their medical education and to explore the essence of their empathy' (Tavakol *et al.* 2009: 306)?

It should be noted that they do not, at any point, consider this alternative. They do not even include a question about 'declining empathy' among the three example questions that they put to the participants during the interviews. I assume that a question of this sort must have been asked at some stage, because the students did actually talk about the decline, or lack of it. But this is a single theme amid a lot of stuff about what the students believe, feel, perceive, or understand about empathy in general. What is baffling is that Tavakol *et al.* (2009) don't home in on 'the decline at the end of Year 3' as a specific research question.[12] Instead, they ask the students to muse about what empathy means, and to talk about their 'empathy experience'.

But if we must talk about 'experience', why does it have to be in this undifferentiated manner? Why is it necessary to ask the students to reflect on 'how they see' empathy in such a general, open-ended fashion when there is a more useful and interesting question staring the authors in the face? Why can't a study of the 'experience of empathy' ask a highly specific question? Why can't it narrow the focus down to one particular aspect of the 'empathy experience'? Why does such a wide-angle lens have to be used?[13] Why can't we just zoom in on what happens at the end of Year 3?

The 'empathy decline' at the end of Year 3 is all the more interesting because, in the discussion section, the authors mention the fact that a few studies have reported no decline (although one of those to which they draw attention was expressly designed to evaluate an empathy-preserving curriculum innovation).[14] 'Clearly, there does not appear to be any consensus on whether empathy declines or is enhanced during medical school' (Tavakol *et al.* 2012: 313–14). However, it is possible that this lack of consensus reflects a more fundamental disagreement about 'the meaning of empathy in the medical education literature' (307).

For example, Tavakol *et al.* first refer to Gladstein (1983), who proposed a two-dimensional model of empathy, 'comprising both cognitive and affective components'; but then note that other authors – and they refer specifically to Hojat *et al.* (2003) – have argued that the affective element is a component of sympathy rather than empathy. But suppose that the two-dimensional model, or something like it, is correct. Isn't it possible that, around the end of Year 3, one of these dimensions declines but the other does not? Suppose, to take just one possibility, that the affective dimension declines, but the cognitive dimension does not? Might that explain the lack of consensus about whether there is a decline at all?

So, at this point, let us *provisionally* take 'the decline in empathy among medical students at the end of Year 3' as the phenomenon to be explained, while allowing for the possibility that this decline affects just one dimension of empathy rather than empathy-as-a-whole.[15] The research question might then be:

> *If there is such a decline, what accounts for it, and which dimension of empathy is affected?*

An answer to this question would be useful in medical education because it would indicate which dimension of empathy was at risk, and suggest ways in which the risk of a decline (in that dimension) could be reduced.

Theoretical considerations: uses of 'empathy'

The specification of the phenomenon and the proposed research question are, at this stage, provisional. There are various things we might come across – including theoretical concepts and research findings – which would prompt a reformulation of both. For although the discussion so far has provided an initial direction, it does not yet represent a platform for the research design. There are at least three conceptual and methodological questions outstanding.

- The first is whether empathy has dimensions (and, if it does, what they are).
- The second is how a decline in empathy (or one of its dimensions) can be measured.
- The third is what sort of data would permit an inference about the explanation of this decline.

The discipline in which we might expect to find the most helpful resources is social psychology, which has an extensive literature on empathy and related concepts (Dovidio *et al.* 2006; Decety and Ickes 2009; Decety 2014). One striking feature of Tavakol *et al.* (2012) is that it makes hardly any reference to this literature. There are only two references to Decety and Ickes (2009), both of them in passing; and there is no discussion of any of the chapters by contributing authors. Yet the first chapter of this book could not be more relevant: 'These things called empathy: eight related but distinct phenomena' (Batson 2009).

It is worth observing, parenthetically, that this material is not difficult to track down. You do not need to be particularly familiar with the literature. When I inserted the keywords 'empathy social psychology' in Google Scholar, the edited book by Decety and Ickes was the fourth hit, and was comfortably the most recent contribution on the first page of hits (the next most recent was 2001). It is,

I would say, the most obvious place to start. Moreover, given that Tavakol *et al.* were obviously aware that 'there is a lack of consensus on the meaning of empathy in the medical literature' (the first sentence of their paper), one would have thought that a careful reading of Batson's chapter would have been a priority.

Batson argues that the word 'empathy' is 'currently applied to more than half a dozen phenomena'. That is to say, he does not distinguish between different 'dimensions' of empathy; rather, he identifies eight distinct things the word is used to refer to in the psychology literature. These are 'not elements, aspects, facets, or components of a single thing that is empathy'. Instead, each is 'a conceptually distinct, stand-alone psychological state'. Further, each of these states 'has been called by names other than empathy' (Batson 2009: 3). As a consequence, and as Batson notes, 'opportunities for disagreement abound'.[16]

The eight psychological states that Batson (4–8) identifies are:

i   Knowing another person's internal state, including his or her thoughts and feelings
ii Adopting the posture or matching the neural responses of an observed other
iii Coming to feel as another person feels
iv Intuiting or projecting oneself into another's situation
v   Imagining how another is thinking and feeling
vi Imagining how one would think and feel in the other's place
vii Feeling distress at witnessing another person's suffering
viii Feeling for another person who is suffering

It is important to recognise the various distinctions that are being made here. Let 'P' be the person who is in a particular psychological state. Let 'R' be the person who is responding to P.

State (i) is a *cognitive* state. R comes to know, or understand, what P's psychological state is. This may result from close observation, or analysis, or asking P relevant questions. Achieving this cognitive state does not require R to have any particular affective state; nor does it imply that she will develop one as a result of achieving the cognitive state.

States (iii), (vii) and (viii) are *affective* states, but they are all different. In (iii), R experiences the same emotion as P, or a very similar one. In (vii), R feels emotional distress at P's suffering, but she does not experience the same emotion as P. In (viii), R feels concern for P. Baton calls this 'empathic concern'. It is an emotional state of R, but it is not the same as P's emotion; nor does personal distress (on R's part) figure in it.

States (iv), (v) and (vi) are *imaginative* states. In (iv), R imagines what it would be like to be in the kind of situation that P is in. In (v), R imagines what it must be like to be, specifically, P in this situation. In (vi), R imagines what she, R, would think and feel if she were in P's place. Each of these states involves imagination, but what is imagined varies. In (iv), it is somebody-in-this-kind-of-situation. In (v), it is P-in-this-situation. In (vi), it is R-in-this-situation.

State (ii) is a *mimetic* state. R's response to P imitates (in some sense, in some respect) P's state. The mechanism here may be behavioural or neural. Behaviourally, R might imitate P's facial expression or posture. Neurally, if R perceives P in a particular situation, R's neural state will automatically (it is said) come to match P's neural state. In either case, R will not necessarily be conscious of her response as a form of imitation.

This, I think, is an illuminating analysis. In particular, the idea that these are all different states, rather than dimensions of the same state, is a significant one. One consequence of this idea is that being in x state does not necessarily entail being in y state. For example:

State (i) does not entail state (iii).

You might know that P feels emotion E, but that does not entail that you feel E yourself. Similarly:

State (vi) does not entail state (i)

You might have a sense of how *you* would feel in the other person's place, but that does not mean that you know how *she* is feeling.

State (viii) does not entail state (vii)

Empathic concern does not require that you, personally, feel any emotional *distress*.

At any rate, suppose that Batson's analysis, or something approximating to it, is correct. It follows that you cannot invite a group of respondents to talk about 'how they see empathy' because they might all interpret the word as referring to a different state. Tavakol *et al.* do recognise that some of their student respondents appear to have sympathy rather than empathy in mind, though it is far from clear what they think the difference is. However, Batson's analysis implies that the situation might be more complicated than mistaking sympathy for empathy. Some of the respondents might have state (vii) in mind, others state (vi). Some might be thinking of state (i), others might be thinking of state (iii). Indeed, it's possible that the same student might be thinking of different states during different parts of the interview. She might, for example, have state (i) in mind during one part of the interview, and state (iii), or state (vii), or state (viii) during another part. Tavakol *et al.* have no way of knowing.

Interestingly, the student has no way of knowing either. How many of us differentiate the various states that 'empathy' can refer to while we are actually using the word? Not many of us, I would think. Before reading Batson's chapter, I found myself struggling to pin down the difference between 'empathy' and 'sympathy', and certainly did not know that 'empathy' is used (by psychologists) to refer to any one of eight distinct states. I doubt I'm the only one. If I'm not, it's quite possible that individual students were referring to different 'empathy' states during different parts of the interview, and never realised this.

In the context of medical education and the 'decline of empathy', Batson's analysis suggests one very important question. If there is a decline in empathy during Year 3, which of these eight states is it that declines? Possibly all of them; but this seems a bit unlikely. So which states decline, and which don't? Are some of them even enhanced? If so, which? It would not be difficult to formulate a hypothesis. For example, perhaps state (vii) declines, while state (viii) remains stable, and state (i) is enhanced. This is a hypothesis that could be tested, and a qualitative study might lead to the construction of a model.

I'll return to this possibility in a moment. First, we need to look at a methodological issue: how empathy is measured.

Methodological considerations: measuring empathy

How do we know that there is a decline of empathy in Year 3? We are taking this decline, provisionally, as the phenomenon to be explained, but on what basis? There are, in fact, several studies that have suggested that a decline in empathy takes place during undergraduate and graduate medical education (Hojat *et al.* 2004; Sherman and Cramer 2005; Chen *et al.* 2007; Newton *et al.* 2008). However, the paper which Tavakol *et al.* refer to, and which has most citations, is Hojat *et al.* (2009), so I will focus on that.

Hojat *et al.* (2009) employed a measure called the Jefferson Scale of Physician Empathy (JSPE), which, as its name suggests, was devised for use specifically with physicians. In this particular study, they used a version of it, JSPE(S), designed expressly for medical students, and worded accordingly. The JSPE(S) incorporates 20 Likert-style items, each of which is scored from +1 to +7. The score for any individual, therefore, ranges from 20 (low empathy) to 140 (high empathy).

Hojat *et al.* (2002) carried out a factor analysis to establish factor loadings for each item. Three factors were identified. The first was 'perspective taking, the core ingredient of empathy'. The second factor was 'compassionate care'. The third was a residual factor (involving only two items): 'ability to stand in the patients' shoes'. I suspect these factors are misnamed. The first is a cognitive factor, referring to an understanding of the patient's psychological state rather than perspective taking as such. The second is an affective factor, referring to the significance (or not) of emotion (primarily the patient's, but also the physician's). The third is perspective taking, referring to the difficulty of seeing things from the patient's point of view.

The measure was administered to two cohorts (2002 and 2004) of students at a single medical school in the US. In each case, the first administration was at the beginning of the students' first year; subsequent administrations were at the end of the first, second, third and fourth years (five administrations in all). To summarise the findings: the mean empathy score, as measured by the JSPE(S), remained stable at about 115 until the end of Year 2 (three administrations), but declined at the end of Year 3 to about 109. This does not look like an enormous drop,[17] but it is statistically significant, and is sufficient to prompt speculation about what accounts for it.

The 20 items of the JSPE make interesting reading. They include:

A   I try to understand what is going on in my patients' minds by paying attention to their nonverbal cues and body language.
B   I try to imagine myself in my patients' shoes when providing care to them.
C   I try to think like my patients in order to render better care.
D   I do not allow myself to be touched by intense emotional relationships among my patients and their family members.
E   My understanding of my patients' feelings gives them a sense of validation that is therapeutic in its own right.
F   I have a good sense of humor that I think contributes to a better clinical outcome.

In Batson's terms, these six items represent at least four different states. The first four can be assigned to the following Batson categories:

A   state (i)
B   state (iv)
C   state (v)
D   state (vii)[18]

What about the remaining two? E is presumably state (i), but no Batson category appears to fit F. It is perhaps intended to reflect the 'communication' aspect of empathy, which Hojat *et al.* (2002) include in their definition. However, E and F have something in common that A, B, C and D do not share. They both refer to *outcomes*: '...gives them a sense of validation that is therapeutic', and '...contributes to a better clinical outcome'.

But the JSPE is supposedly an instrument that measures empathy, the extent to which the physician or student is empathetic or not. E and F are about something else entirely: the belief that empathy (on some understanding) is therapeutic. However, there is quite clearly a difference between *being* empathetic and *believing* that empathy is therapeutic. On my reading, no less than seven of the JSPE items go beyond a measure of empathy, and include belief in its effectiveness (for example: 'Empathy is a therapeutic skill without which my success as a health care provider would be limited').

I am not sure I understand why an instrument intended to measure the ability to empathise incorporates items that assess the respondent's belief in the effectiveness of empathy. Obviously, you can believe that empathy is therapeutic, but not be particularly empathetic yourself. So if seven out of 20 items assess 'belief in effectiveness', it's not clear how good the JSPE can be at measuring the 'ability to empathise'.

At any rate, the 20 items of the JSPE cover at least six of Batson's categories (with seven items adding belief-in-effectiveness to empathetic-attitude). It would have been interesting if the longitudinal study of medical students (Hojat *et al.* 2009) had included some analysis of individual items. Given that the decline in empathy at the end of Year 3 is relatively small (115 to 109), it is possible that a handful of items are responsible for it. Unfortunately, however, Hojat *et al.* stick with mean scores for the overall scale, and do not even break the findings down into the three factors that they had previously identified.

For the qualitative researcher, then, there are interesting questions about the decline in empathy at the end of Year 3. For example:

*   Is the decline explained by the fact that students begin to differentiate the various states that can be called 'empathy'?
*   Do they continue to acknowledge the necessity of understanding their patients' feelings, while recognising that they cannot afford to become distressed?
*   Do they distinguish between 'feeling what the patient feels' and 'feeling for a person who is suffering', recognising that the latter does not have to be accompanied by the former?
*   Do they realise that understanding somebody's internal state does not necessarily mean that they must be able to project themselves into that person's situation?

If we are to answer these questions, and evaluate the implications for medical education, we need to be clear about how interviewing students can help to explain why a decline in empathy occurs – or, rather, why there is a change in one (or more) of the states to which the word 'empathy' is used to refer.

Decline in empathy: interviewing strategy

This discussion prompts an obvious question. Would it not be a good idea to forget about 'empathy', with its definitional complexity, and home in on specific skills, abilities and attitudes? Should we not abandon the assumption of 'one word, one thing' (note 16) and, instead of asking whether there is a 'decline in empathy', evaluate the extent to which there is a decline in a particular skill (understanding what the patient is feeling, for example) or a particular affective state (a certain emotional response to the patient's situation)? If we were to take this line, Batson's categories would be undeniably helpful.

At this point, all sorts of possibilities open up. If we were not to restrict the methodological options to interviewing, we could consider a behavioural study. This would have the advantage of avoiding self-report (whether in quantitative or qualitative form) and the cognitive biases to which it is subject. Ideas for such a study can be found in the same collection as that in which the Batson chapter appears.[19] For example, Ickes (2009) describes several behavioural tests of the ability to 'read' other people's thoughts and feeling.

For the qualitative researcher, however, adopting these behavioural measures would pose a problem, or possibly two. First, interviews would have reduced importance, since the question 'Is there a decline in people-reading ability or not?' would be decided by a behavioural indicator. Second, this alternative would imply a longitudinal design, administering the test at different stages of medical education to determine whether there was a decline in people-reading ability at the end of Year 3. This might require time and resources not available to some qualitative researchers, especially postgraduates.

In the rest of this section, therefore, I will focus on what might be achieved with interviews, conducted on a non-longitudinal basis.

Let's take Batson's categories as a jumping-off point. First, the categories can probably be pruned. For one thing, state (ii) ('Adopting the posture or matching the neural response of another person') is not something respondents will be able to comment on. They will have no idea about neural responses, and it is unlikely that they will be aware of their own posture and facial expressions when they are working with patients. For another, state (iv) and state (v) are not easy to discriminate: even Batson's description is rather ambiguous about the difference. But we can certainly distinguish between the *cognitive* state (i), the *feeling* states (iii, vii and viii), and the *imaginative* states (iv, v, and vi). So interviewing medical students using these superordinate categories as a reference point is feasible.

Next, the 'broad question' approach of Tavakol *et al.* won't be effective if we are seeking to understand what kind of shift occurs during Year 3. Given the specific nature of the enquiry we're considering, it is absolutely necessary that the respondents are briefed on the purpose of the research before the interview begins. They should be informed about the studies indicating that a decline in empathy occurs, and told that the aim of the interview is to explore their own thoughts about this, as students who have recently had experience of the third year. They should also be introduced to the superordinate classification: the cognitive, affective and imaginative categories to which seven of Batson's states can be assigned. If this is done, the interview can proceed on the basis of:

> This is some previous research, this is what we think, this is what we're wondering about.... Now, as somebody who has recently been in Year 3, how does that reflect your experience?[20]

So the respondent would be informed that the interviewer is interested in the doctor/patient relationship, and the various things that are said about it. In particular, she is interested in what students think about the following questions: To what extent should a doctor be trying to understand the patient's thoughts and feelings? How important is this, given the primary tasks of diagnosis and treatment? What should the doctor feel (or not feel) themselves? How far should a doctor be trying to imagine what this situation is like for the patient? Does any of this affect empathic concern? And so on.

As with any form of qualitative interviewing, slightly broader questions can be asked first. For example:

> To what extent, if at all, have your thoughts about practising medicine, and in particular the doctor/patient relationship, changed over the past year?

As far as you can tell, has working directly with patients during the last year had any impact on your thoughts about the doctor/patient relationship?

If you *are* conscious of any change in your thinking about the doctor/patient relationship, are there any particular situations or cases that might have prompted that?

More specific questions might include:

In general, how much interest do you take in the patient's thoughts and feelings about what is happening to him or her?

Does this vary from patient to patient? Or is there a pattern that applies to everybody?

Do you make any attempt to assess what the patient might be thinking or feeling? If so, on what basis? What information helps with this?

If you do try to gauge the patient's thoughts and feelings, what sort of difference does that make to how to manage the consultation?

How good would you say you are at assessing the patient's thoughts and feelings?

Has this ability developed during the past year? If so, how and why?

Is this a skill which you feel the need to develop further? If so, in what respects? If not, why do you feel you have gone as far as you can or are prepared to?

Are you conscious of having emotions yourself when you're working with a patient?

If so, what kinds of emotions/feelings? Are they limited to general concern for the patient's welfare, or do you ever experience distress yourself?

Are you conscious of any limits you impose on your concern for the patient's welfare?

Is it possible, do you think, to care too much about the patient?

How far is it true, do you think, that doctors need to protect themselves from feeling too much? Why is that?

To what extent do you try to keep your feelings under control?

Do you ever try to imagine what the situation must be like for the patient, or what you personally would feel if you were in that situation?

Is it more appropriate to imagine what *you* would feel in this situation, or to imagine what this particular *patient* is feeling?

Does this vary from patient to patient? If so, what kinds of patient would prompt you to do this?

The key question, relative to the research question, is:

To what extent have your views on this changed or developed over the past year? What do you think prompted these changes?

A few brief comments on this list.

First, it is by no means comprehensive. Indeed, it barely scratches the surface of possible questions that could be asked using the Batson categories as a guide.

Second, the 'key' question can/should be asked as a follow-up to any of the others.

Third, none of the questions mentions empathy. Rather, Batson's categories are employed to pose more specific questions, permitting (or encouraging) the respondents to discriminate between the states that the categories refer to. In effect, the researcher operationalises the term 'empathy', instead of delegating responsibility for operationalising it to the respondent (which is what Tavakol *et al.* do).

Fourth, the questions would need piloting. In particular, alternative words would have to be evaluated. Is there a difference between 'develop' and 'change'? Or do students regard them as synonymous? Do students recognise a distinction between 'emotion' and 'feeling'? Would 'evaluate' or 'judge' be clearer than 'assess'? Does the use of 'thoughts', 'views', or 'attitudes' make any difference to the response? Is there a difference between 'impact' and 'effect'? Do the students think in terms of the 'doctor/patient relationship', or is some other concept a better fit with how they conceptualise their role? And so on.

It will not be clear, prior to piloting, whether any of these terms is understood by the respondents in the way the researcher intends.[21] For example, it is not clear whether the respondents would identify with 'changed' (as in 'Have your thoughts changed?'), or whether they would be more likely to identify with 'developed' (or 'moved on', or 'progressed'). Which of these words would be more likely to prompt the kind of reflection that the interviewer seeks? Or would they all have a similar effect?

Fifth, piloting would also be required to determine whether these questions (and the locations in which the interviews take place) permit honest answers, or whether they encourage the respondents to succumb to social desirability bias – to say what they think someone involved in medical education would want to hear.[22]

The proposed interviewing strategy may be rather different from PQR, but it is closely related to other approaches (especially that of Pawson and Tilley 1997). Compared with the strategy of Tavakol *et al.*, it has a much better chance of generating data capable of explaining the phenomenon.

Decline in empathy: analysis

How would an analysis of the data generated by questions of the kind listed above proceed? Well, in the first place, the analyst could determine the extent to which the Batson categories applied to the students' responses. It is, of course, quite possible that further distinctions, or perhaps different ones, might have to be made.

For example, it might be necessary to distinguish between different responses to questions about state (i). On what basis do the medical students (by the time they reach Year 4 or 5) acquire knowledge of the patient's thoughts and feelings, and to what extent does this change or develop during Year 3? The methods that students refer to might include: asking relevant questions (directed to the patient and/or the family), observation of behaviour and body language, observation of facial expressions, intuition, study of medical notes and records, or some permutation. Conceivably, too, a student might report that her skill in one or more of these methods might be enhanced during the course of the year. This is still self-report, and such claims should be treated cautiously. If a student claimed that she had learned to interpret facial expressions (for example) more accurately, this should probably be treated with circumspection. If, however, she could support the claim with a more detailed account of *how* she learned to do this, that would be more persuasive than a bare and unelaborated statement. Moreover, if combined with an admission that, in spite of her enhanced ability to read facial expressions, she is still unable to interpret body language effectively, her account might carry even greater conviction.

As I have already suggested, it is possible that one or more Batson-states might decline, even while one or more of the other Batson-states remain stable or are enhanced. So, for example, some students might report an increased ability to 'read' patients but, equally, a greater reluctance to embrace certain feelings. We might suppose that this is particularly likely with states (iii) and (vii). Students might decide that it is not advisable to let oneself feel personal distress, or too much distress, when confronted with a patient who is suffering (state vii). This might be for either or both of two related reasons: first, it produces too much emotional wear and tear on the student; second, it interferes with her ability to think objectively and constructively about treatment. Additionally, (or alternatively), students might decide that it is not necessary to 'feel as the patient feels' in order to have some understanding of what the patient is going through. You can understand that the patient is experiencing distress or anxiety without experiencing distress or anxiety yourself. Moreover, taking the patient's perspective in *this* sense – having the same emotions as the patient – might well be thought distracting and counterproductive.

In summary, it is possible that the student's ability to 'read' patients might be enhanced at the same time as she decides to dial down on feelings of distress herself, or desists from her attempts to experience the patient's own emotions.

It is worth adding that this 'dialling down' on states (iii) and (vii) is compatible with continuing to 'feel for another person who is suffering' – that is, state (viii). You can continue to experience, and express, empathic concern for the patient even if you distance yourself from personal distress and attempts to 'feel what the patient feels'. So one possibility is that (a) the students' 'mindreading' ability increases, (b) their inclination to embrace distress and/or engage with the patient's emotions declines, but (c) their concern for the patient remains stable. If something of this sort were true, then any talk about a 'decline in empathy' at the end of Year 3 would be simplistic.

Of course, this is all speculative. I am not offering a view about what this sort of study would show. I am suggesting how such a study could be carried out, and how the data it produced could be analysed. However, the Tavakol *et al.*

paper does contain hints that something along these lines might be correct. According to the authors, 'participants had different experiences of and explanations for the decline or enhancement of empathy'. To illustrate this, they quote one student who says (311):

> I think now that I've come to the end of medical school, it affects me less emotionally ... I felt very emotional a lot of the time dealing with breaking bad news, watching people die, watching people go through horrible operations, watching people get sick, dealing with their families. That used to affect me and it affects me less now, but it's not because I don't feel it, it's because I don't let it affect my emotions as much.

The focus here is very much on feelings and emotions. There has been some dialling down ('it affects me less emotionally ... it affects me less now'), although it is not immediately obvious what the student means when she says: 'it's not because I don't feel it, it's because I don't let it affect my emotions as much'. She is clearly making an important distinction, but what she says is not completely transparent. One possibility is that she is referring to the difference between state (viii) (feeling for another person who is suffering) and state (vii) (feeling distress at witnessing that suffering). This might explain the statement that she *feels* it (state viii) but doesn't let it *affect her emotions* as much (state vii).

She may, of course, mean something different, but it is difficult to tell because she does not really have the vocabulary to spell out exactly what she has in mind. If the interviewer had made use of Batson's categories, or if she had introduced some other theoretical perspective to the discussion, it is possible that this respondent might have been able to express herself more precisely.[23]

Later on the same page, Tavakol *et al.* quote a different student:

> I understand a bit more about the conditions and I know how they affect patients ... I think it is to do with education as well, because once you've understood the different ways patients can be affected and you've seen patients being affected. Because obviously in the first year we didn't see many patients anyway.

Unlike the previous respondent, this student emphasises understanding ('I understand ... I know ... once you've understood') and does not, at least in this passage, refer to her own emotions. According to her account, this particular ability – to understand how various illness conditions affect patients – has been enhanced. It has certainly not declined. It would obviously be interesting to know what this respondent would say about the management of her own emotions, and whether this too had changed as a result of seeing patients. Would she say the same as the previous respondent, or something different? It is clearly possible that the enhancement of her ability to understand has been accompanied by the moderation of her feelings. So the speculative analysis sketched above is not implausible.

Tavakol *et al.* suggest that 'participants had different experiences of and explanations for the decline or enhancement of empathy'; but the quoted extracts are consistent with students recognising that they had improved their 'mindreading' ability, while observing that they had curtailed their feeling responses.

At one point, however, Tavakol *et al.* do notice this possibility. Having repeated that the participants had 'contrasting experiences with respect to the decline or enhancement of empathy', they suggest:

> Perhaps these comments also demonstrate that whereas students may experience a more affective or emotional type of empathy at the beginning of their studies, their focus tends to shift towards a more intellectual or cognitive version of empathy as training progresses.
>
> (311)

But they can't have it both ways. *Either* different students had 'different experiences of empathy', *or* they began to differentiate between cognitive states and affective states. Tavakol *et al.* generally adopt the first of these alternatives.

So there are reasons to suppose that increased 'mindreading' ability might be a feature of Year 3, but that it is accompanied by a moderation of the more intense emotional responses (even if students continue to feel sympathy and concern for their patients). In fact, it is likely to be rather more complex than this. Elsewhere, Tavakol *et al.* refer to 'empathetic behaviour', 'demonstrating empathy', 'rapport building', and other expressions suggesting that the students talked about how they communicate with patients as an 'aspect of empathy'. It is possible, then, that 'empathise' in the students' usage might refer, not just to cognitive, affective and imaginative capacities, but also to behavioural ones. There are hints in the published excerpts that 'displaying empathy' may be another ability that is enhanced in Year 3 instead of declining.

There is still one question outstanding. Let us suppose that Year 3 sees a progressive differentiation of cognitive, affective, imaginative, and behavioural states. Cognitive and imaginative abilities improve, while the inclination to engage with intense feelings declines. At the same time, empathic concern for the patient remains stable. The question is: why does this occur?

Empathy: a 'how possibly' model

A study of the kind I proposed earlier could get closer to answering this question than the Tavakol *et al.* PQR study. Once again, however, there are some hints about the relevant mechanisms in their paper. One is the fact that in Year 3 students see more patients. As the student quoted above notes, 'in the first year we didn't see many patients anyway'. Another is the opportunity to observe experienced doctors in clinical environments, some of whom 'don't have great empathy skills'. So, for example:

If you've got a team with a doctor who doesn't like that kind of thing, then the rest of the team tend to follow suit. I think it's difficult for medical students to ... take into account the emotions of the patient if they're in an unsupportive environment.

(Tavakol *et. al* 2012: 311)

These comments suggest that the more intensive encounter with both patients and doctors from Year 3 onwards has an impact on the students' attitude to empathy. The encounter with patients provides an opportunity to develop one's 'mindreading' abilities,[24] but also provides an incentive to subdue the personal emotions that these encounters can precipitate. The encounter with doctors can, in some cases, inhibit the *expression* of empathic concern (and may create an additional incentive to down-regulate personal feelings).[25] This is probably an effect of imitation, conformity, or social pressure.[26]

Interestingly, this explanation (or sketch of an explanation) is different from the one mentioned briefly by Tavakol *et al.* towards the beginning of their paper: 'An explanation suggested for this decline is that the focus on a biomedical model undermines the biopsychosocial model, which includes the patient's psychological and emotional needs' (the authors reference Spiro 2009). Competing explanations could, of course, be tested by research of the kind I have been proposing. However, one puzzling aspect of the account attributed to Spiro is that it fails to explain why the 'undermining' occurs specifically in Year 3. Presumably, it would be a cumulative effect of several years' exposure to the biomedical model, and would have nothing directly to do with encountering more patients and doctors in clinical environments.

Putting the fragmentary data from Tavakol *et al.* together with the 'dialling down' metaphor, Batson's states, and some plausible mechanisms from social psychology – 'some bits of theories, some bits of empirical evidence and a metaphor' (Morrison and Morgan 1999: 13) – we can outline a preliminary, 'how-possibly' model (Figure 7.2) of what happens in Year 3 of medical school, at least in Nottingham (where the Tavakol *et al.* study was conducted).

The student begins, we can suppose, with a generally positive but undifferentiated attitude towards something called 'empathy'. Since there is no consensus among psychologists about how to define the term, and if Batson is right in saying that it is applied to several different states, there is no reason to think that medical students are any clearer about what it refers to.

Year 3 exposure to both patients and doctors in clinical environments prompts a change, the underlying dynamic of which is progressive differentiation. This will rarely be explicit, or expressed in a nuanced vocabulary, but it will be apparent in how the student talks (and more so, presumably, in how she acts). This differentiation will involve an implicit distinction between cognitive and imaginative capacities, personal emotions, behavioural expression of these emotions, and empathic concern for the patient. As a consequence of various social psychological mechanisms (notes 23, 24, 25), the cognitive capacity ('mindreading') will generally speaking be enhanced, personal

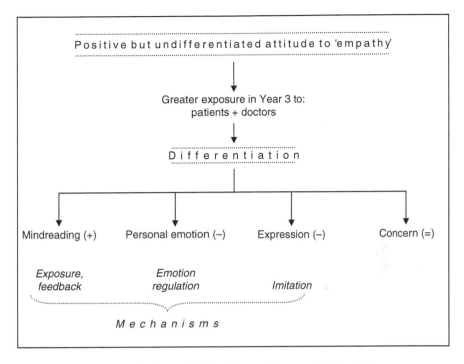

Figure 7.2 Empathy decline in medical students: a 'how possibly' model.

emotion will be down-regulated, and the open expression of sympathetic concern will be inhibited.

This, as I have said, is only a sketch of a model. However, it is a model that could be tested, refined and elaborated by interview-based qualitative research – provided that the interviews concerned focused on the concrete details of the students' reactions to Year 3. Theory drawn from social psychology, together with research findings from other relevant sub-disciplines, is unavoidable in the planning, conduct, and analysis of such a study.

Overview: bits of theory

This has been an extended discussion of a research possibility arising from the Tavakol *et al.* paper, in which I have shown how: (a) a topic can be converted into a phenomenon-to-be-explained by reference to established findings; (b) useful theory from a relevant discipline, in this case social psychology, can be incorporated into the design and conduct of a qualitative study; (c) previous findings and selected elements from social psychological theory can be used to construct a 'how-possibly' model capable of explaining the phenomenon.

It would not have been possible to condense this discussion into a simple recipe, at least not without a considerable loss of information. Instead, I have tried to illustrate the thinking process that informs this kind of research, taking the reader through a case study based on a published paper in order to show that there are constructive alternatives to PQR. If I had more space, I would provide further examples.

Inevitably, I've been critical of the Tavakol *et al.* study itself. But my criticisms reflect what I have said in the rest of the book about PQR in general, and I could have given virtually any published PQR study the same sort of treatment. Buried somewhere in PQR discussions, there is nearly always a clue to what the alternative might have looked like: a study aimed at constructing a model capable of explaining a phenomenon, rather than a study designed to explore a topic by asking people to talk, indiscriminately, about their experiences. So in this case an accusation of cherry-picking would be beside the point. The primary purpose of this chapter has not been to criticise, but to take the published paper as a starting point, and see what kind of study could have been carried out instead.

I should emphasise, however, that there are other possibilities inherent in the Tavakol *et al.* paper. I do not pretend that the sort of study I have outlined is the best, or only possible, option. The phenomenon that stood out for me was the third year 'decline'. Others might have homed in on an alternative. Nor do I imagine that the model I have suggested is the last word on the 'decline' issue. If a study of the kind I have sketched were actually carried out, it might culminate in a model considerably at variance with this one. The point of the case study is not to get the model right, but to show how it can be arrived at.

The case study is obviously intended to be the antithesis of PQR. It does not take the axiom of resident meaning as its premise, and it makes extensive use of 'imported' theories. The interpretation of the data taken from Tavakol *et al.* is not based on the idea that the 'meaning of the phenomenon' is somehow contained (but hidden) in the interview transcripts; rather, it is based explicitly on theories drawn from social psychology (Batson, Ickes, Marangoni, Gross, Asch, and the secondary literature devoted to these authors). The contrast with Giorgi, van Manen and SFL could not be more apparent.

It has been suggested to me that a theory-based approach requires too great an immersion in disciplines beyond health care. How many postgraduate nursing students can confidently draw on a background in social psychology, for example? The advantage of PQR (and other QRAS approaches) is precisely that this kind of immersion is deemed to be unnecessary: people's experiences can be elicited independently of theory, and data can be analysed by looking for themes that 'emerge' from the data itself.

However, the reference to 'immersion' considerably overstates what is required. In working through the empathy example, I drew on material that took no more than a couple of evenings' Googling to find. I was already aware of the Decety and Ickes volume, but had not studied it in any detail; and I was broadly familiar with the work of Asch. However, the rest was new, discovered in the course of Google Scholar searches, with (initially) only the Tavakol *et al.* paper as a guide.

For example, it occurred to me that social psychologists must have investigated the conditions in which empathic accuracy is enhanced. Marangoni *et al.* (1995) was the fifth hit on the first page of a Google Scholar search. Similarly, when I found myself talking about the possibility of students 'dialling down' on personal emotion during Year 3, it occurred to me that, again, the process must have been studied, and that there was probably a better, theoretically informed, expression than the colloquial 'dialling down'. Instead of inserting the search terms 'dialling down emotion' in Google Scholar, I tried 'reduce emotion' and then, more in hope than expectation, 'reduce down emotion' (since the 'down' bit struck me as a compelling image). This brought me (sixth hit on the first page) to another paper by Gross, in which the expression 'down-regulate emotion' was used. A scan of Gross's other publications led to Gross (2002), which seemed to be exactly what I was looking for.

The design stage was even more straightforward. Having turned up Decety and Ickes almost immediately, I spent the rest of the evening reading the Batson chapter and thinking about its implications. The next evening, I spent a bit of time considering how one might construct an interview schedule, drawing on Batson's work. Discovering that he had also published a monograph in the same year (Batson 2011), I had a quick look at the Google Books version of it, to see whether it included any additional material I could use. (It did, but I decided not to introduce it into this discussion, because it would have made the chapter even longer.)

Of course, if I were to undertake a study of 'third year decline in empathy' for real, rather than as a case study exercise, I would read far more widely. I would dig further into the literature, examine alternative theories, look at a wider range of mechanisms. However, I don't think I would have to do more than a postgraduate student could do, or should be expected to. What I hope to have shown, in any case, is that promising theoretical leads can be retrieved rather quickly and that, by reading only a handful of papers and chapters, it is possible to accumulate sufficient material to construct a plausible (but, as I have said, not definitive) model.

So full immersion in social psychology, or any other discipline, is not required. All that is necessary is a good search strategy, a willingness to read unfamiliar stuff, and an ability to make connections. None of these is beyond the ability or ambitions of a postgraduate student, though they do need a certain amount of practice to develop them fully.

I would claim that the results of a theoretically informed explaining-the-phenomenon study are far more likely to be useful than a theory-averse, exploring-the-topic study. Suppose, for example, that the model of 'empathy decline' sketched above were to be supported by additional evidence. What would it imply about medical education and how to improve it? In the first instance, I think, it would imply that there is no cause for panic (especially since the fall in JSPE scores at the end of the third year is not dramatic).

Exposure to patients and doctors in clinical environments is almost bound to prompt an adjustment in the students' thoughts about the doctor/patient relationship, and if the model represents this adjustment accurately, finding a means of combating the 'cynicism [which] develops progressively during their training' (Hojat *et al.* 2009: 1185) is hardly an urgent priority. Of course, this is not to argue that communication skills, role play, humanities, and so on should be dropped from the curriculum. It is to say, instead, that most students seem to regulate their empathy-related states quite successfully in the face of clinical experience, even if their 'empathy' scores decrease by a small but statistically significant amount.

Beyond this initial conclusion, several suggestions might be made. One is to prepare the students for the adjustment, possibly by introducing them to the different Batson-states that the term 'empathy', in its undifferentiated sense, runs together. Recognising that down-regulating emotion is both predictable and legitimate, that it is not incompatible with continuing to feel empathic concern for patients, and that it does not necessarily prevent the development of cognitive and imaginative capacities, might give the students a better understanding of the process of differentiation itself, and might help them to negotiate their way through it. A second suggestion is to ensure that students are given regular feedback on their 'mindreading' skills, since the evidence suggests that this enhances those skills significantly. A third is to find some way of intervening in an 'unsupportive environment', if that is inhibiting the expression of empathic concern. 'Following suit' may be a familiar mechanism; but, as Asch's experiments show, it is a far from inevitable one.

The 'empathy decline' model has practical implications because it is the outcome of a study that sets out to *explain* a phenomenon. You can do something with an understanding of cause and effect that you can't do with 'meaning' or 'essence'. The discussion section of Tavakol *et al.* begins by noting that 'in terms of the essence of empathy, this study reveals that students feel that empathy is fundamental to medical care'; and goes on to tell us what other views the ten students have on the subject. I don't know what the practical implications of this conclusion are: a handful of students at a single university have a range of not-entirely-consistent thoughts about empathy, and these thoughts represent 'the essence of their understanding of empathy'. I hesitate to ask 'So what?', but that is the question lurking in my mind.

'What practical use can I make of this?' is the most important question in health-related research. If it cannot be answered convincingly, it is not clear what value the study in question can have.

The undecided: concluding thought

At the beginning of this book I suggested that my primary constituency consisted of the undecided, the waverers, the curious, the provisionally attracted, the secretly baffled, the at-a-loss. I stated that my aim was to give them reasons for pausing before they settle on the PQR approach, and that I would provide an outline of a more promising alternative.

Most of this chapter has been devoted to that outline; but I will close with a reminder of the reasons for pausing. They are contained, largely, in Chapters 3, 4 and 6. Study the three methodological texts, read those three chapters, and then decide whether the procedures advocated by Giorgi, van Manen and SFL can be followed. Do you understand why Giorgi makes minor changes in the syntax or introduces trivial synonyms? Do you understand why his amendments are 'more revelatory of the psychological aspect of the lived-through experience' (Chapter 3)? Do you understand how van Manen gets from the narrative of Robert's mother to his Pauline essay on hope? Do you understand why he associates dropping a child off at school with *Sophie's Choice* and *Hansel and Gretel* (Chapter 4)? Do you understand why SFL believe that Keith 'regresses' to being a scolded child when Diane challenges him about the mobile? Do you understand why they change 'finding out' to 'finding', or why they suggest that 'Everyone knew' when Jack describes how he pretended to all his friends that nothing was wrong (Chapter 6)?

If, in all honesty, you can answer 'yes' to these questions, fair enough (though I have no idea how you do it). If, on the other hand, you answer 'no', then your attitude towards PQR may become as sceptical as mine, and you may find yourself wondering whether an alternative, incorporating an explicit appeal to theory, is worth your time and energy. I hope that this last chapter has done something to persuade you that it is.

Notes

1 Widdowson is referring to critical discourse analysis (CDA), not to phenomenology. However, CDA adopts the axiom of resident meaning, just as phenomenology does, so Widdowson's conclusions echo mine. This is particularly noticeable in his comments on instances of CDA practice. In referring to van Dijk (1996), for example, he observes: 'There is nothing at all in the text that warrants these inferences: they are a function of van Dijk's reading of his own pretextual assumptions into it' (105). I have been saying the same kind of thing about SFL and van Manen.

2 I should perhaps repeat an earlier observation. None of what I have said here implies that Giorgi's description of jealousy is necessarily wrong (though I think it is), or that van Manen's understanding of Robert's mother's train of thought is necessarily wrong (*ditto*), or that SFL's interpretation of the HIV interview transcript is necessarily wrong (again *ditto*). The point is rather that, while all three authors officially endorse the axiom of resident meaning, none of them complies with it. Giorgi sticks to the text, but produces no meaning. SFL and van Manen produce meaning, but do not stick to the text. Van Manen and SFL break their own rules. Giorgi obeys the rules, but unwittingly demonstrates their sterility.

3 This is how I understand Heidegger's 'fore-structure of understanding', and in particular 'fore-sight', or *Vorsicht*. The effect of *Vorsicht* is to narrow down the range of possible perspectives I might bring to a topic, text, or batch of data, depending on what interests me at the time. It is important to see that one *brings* a perspective, *Vorsicht*, to interpretation. It is something one adopts for a purpose or, as Heidegger might put it, a for-sake-of-which. 'We approach situations with an eye to what we want to pay specific attention to; we zero in on this or that' (Carman 2003: 213). Heidegger talks of being 'guided', and says that when we come to interpret something in a particular context, 'this is always done under the guidance of a point of view,

which fixes that with regard to which what is understood is to be interpreted' (Heidegger 1962: 191).

This idea is one that PQR writers generally miss. They read the fore-structure of understanding as something internal, something *subjective*. They take it to be the equivalent of a set of preconceptions that the researcher has, and that she may not be aware of. Smith (2007) explicitly equates 'fore-structure' and 'preconceptions', for example, and talks about how he is 'influenced by my preconceptions, shaped by my experience'. He talks of 'acknowledging my preconceptions', 'articulating one's pre-conceptions', and being able to 'see my preconceptions' (6/10). PQR authors typically read Heidegger through a subjectivist prism. The fore-structure of understanding is interpreted as an array of preconceptions in which the researcher is 'imprisoned', unless she is able to identify them through a process of reflection. Instead of a per-spective to be adopted consciously and explicitly, *Vorsicht* is construed as a set of taken-for-granted assumptions, buried in the researcher's head. I discuss the subjec-tivisation of Heidegger in Paley (2014b).

4   Authors such as Miles and Huberman (1994), Silverman (2000), and 6 and Bellamy (2012) do recognise this, of course. I will say more about theories, models and induc-tion later in the chapter.

5   Hacking (2000) is a good introduction to the debate about natural kinds as it pertains to the social sciences. LaPorte (2004) argues that to describe something as a 'natural kind' is to imply that references to it have explanatory value. In other words, if some-thing belongs to a 'natural kind', it must be possible for it to participate in a causal process.

6   For something more up to date, see a recent *Church Times* article: Wyatt (2014). According to the Usual Sunday Attendance statistic, 40 years ago about 3 per cent of the English population attended an Anglican church. The figure is now 1.5 per cent. The Average Weekly Attendance across England in 2012 was 1.05 million. In 2013, it was 1,009,000, a fall of about 4 per cent. The latest figure, as I write, shows that average weekly attendance has fallen below one million for the first time (Sherwood 2016).

7   'Mechanism' and 'mechanical models' are expressions that frighten some people off. They hear the sound of clanking. However, the terms are as benign as 'causation' (see Chapter 2, note 5). They do not entail determinism or automatism – although certain psychological mechanisms do imply that one's reasons for action may be uncon-scious. But that's as scary as it gets. If the consultants who were invited to talk about their own expertise (by Atsalos *et al.* 2014) presented themselves in an impossibly good light, that is not really surprising. As 'self-serving bias', this tendency is an example of a psychological mechanism. And here, 'bias' does not refer to a conscious prejudice or preference (as in: 'he is biased in favour of members of his own family'), but to an unconscious pattern of thought triggered by certain situations. Self-serving bias is the tendency we all have, in a range of circumstances, to exaggerate our own strengths, play down our weaknesses, and edit the stories we tell about ourselves in order to portray ourselves as cleverer, funnier, more competent, and more successful than we really are. For an effective neutralisation of the pejorative associations of 'mental mechanism', see Bechtel (2007).

8   I have updated the amounts. In the actual experiment, subjects were paid $20 (worth over $160 now) or $1.

9   I suspect that cognitive dissonance played a role in the events at Mid Staffordshire NHS Foundation trust between 2005 and 2009, which were the subject of the Francis Report (Francis 2013). My thoughts about how the 'appalling care' at Mid Staffs might have come about are outlined in Paley (2014a). The paper outlines a model of how the 'appalling care' phenomenon could be explained, without resorting to assumptions about 'bad apple' nurses, and without concluding that it is possible to identify people who lack compassion prior to them being trained and entering the

profession. In terms of Craver's distinction (two paragraphs further in the text), this is very much a 'how-possibly' model.

10 Put aside the fact that the sample size in this study is only ten. Overlook the fact that it has not been explained what an 'essence' is. According to the authors, the study reveals ('in terms of the essence of empathy') that students 'feel that empathy is fundamental to medical care'. 'They believe empathy to be a combination of understanding, experience and imagination.' Let us assume, for the sake of argument, that this can be understood to be the essence of *empathy*, as opposed to the essence of teaching, writing, conducting experiments, film-making, architecture, mathematics, or anything else that is a 'combination of understanding, experience and imagination' (almost every kind of thoughtful human activity, in other words). What are we supposed to do with this conclusion? They 'feel that empathy is...'; they 'believe empathy to be...' ('in terms of the essence of empathy'). What decisions do these statements help us to make? What practical implications can be derived from them? What policy questions do they provide an answer to? What puzzles do they resolve? To which van Manen would no doubt reply: 'The question is not: Can we do something with phenomenology? Rather, we should wonder: Can phenomenology do something with us?' (see Chapter 4). It makes you want to bang your head against the wall.

11 Their *Vorhabe*, or 'fore-having', in Heideggerian terms.

12 Or, rather, it's not baffling at all. Their reasoning follows a well-worn groove. Previous studies have used a quantitative approach, which is apparently no good at exploring views and attitudes (even though there is an enormous literature on attitude measures, including implicit attitude measures: Wittenbrink and Schwarz 2007). The individual's social reality cannot be understood from statistical procedures (this is an article of faith: there is no explanation of why not). So an 'inductive, qualitative' approach is adopted instead; and that inevitably means a study of experience. From there to the 'lifeworld' and the 'essential structure of phenomena' is but a short step. A few quick, familiar tropes, and in less than half a page, we have arrived at a 'phenomenological' study, grounded in 'tacit knowledge and the subjectivity of individuals who construct meanings'. The reductionist PQR steamroller flattens everything in its path.

13 The most familiar response is this: asking specific questions imposes the researcher's agenda and concepts on the participant. The participant might not understand 'the phenomenon' in the same way the researcher does, so questions should be kept general, open-ended, minimalist, so as to permit the respondent to talk about the phenomenon in a manner that is salient to her rather than in a manner that is salient to the researcher. This strategy gives the respondent licence to talk about anything that takes her fancy, as long it is broadly related to 'the phenomenon'. But if it is illegitimate to focus the respondents on specific issues – puzzles and problems that have been identified in the research literature – it is little wonder that PQR respondents rarely produce anything that can actually be used. If we need a particular bit of information to solve a particular problem, it is no good inviting participants to wander around the topic as they see fit. They are likely to produce material that is vague, repetitive, and already familiar.

For example, consider the implications of the minimalist approach in the study of a life-threatening illness. If, as a matter of principle, researchers refrain from imposing their own concepts and categories on the respondent; if they avoid specific questions for fear of imposing their own agenda; if they merely invite the participant to talk about his experience 'in his own words', without any clue as to the question they are trying to answer, then the respondent is likely to discuss whatever comes to mind. As a result, he will almost certainly cover the same ground as other respondents in comparable studies: the shock of the diagnosis, the difficulty of coming to terms with a life-limiting disease, the stress of living with the condition, the embarrassment or discomfort of certain symptoms, the psychological consequences, the attempt to maintain a semblance of normality and independence, disruption of ordinary life, the support of family, friends or health professionals, and so on. I certainly do not want to underplay the horror, the anxiety, the misery and, in some cases, the tragedy conveyed by these stories. But, in research terms, they are excessively familiar. The minimalist approach is, in effect, a device for reproducing the same basic narrative over and over again.

14   It is unclear why these 'no decline' studies are not referred to in the introductory part of the paper. Nor is it clear – because their discussion is rather confusing – whether the authors believe that there is a decline (or not). However, anybody who wants to promote empathy-enhancing, or empathy-preserving, initiatives in medical education has an incentive to believe that a decline is likely in the absence of any curriculum innovation. For example:

> Maintaining empathy during the third year of medical school is possible through educational intervention. A curriculum that includes safe, protected time for third-year students to discuss their reactions to patient care situations during clerkships may have contributed to the preservation of empathy.
>
> (Rosenthal *et al.* 2011: 350)

This is the evaluation study referred to by Tavakol *et al.* in the discussion section.

15   I am not, of course, suggesting that this is the only 'empathy' phenomenon that might be studied. I am sure there are many more. However, given the literature to which Tavakol *et al.* refer, it is the one that most obviously suggests itself.

16   Many authors seem to hold an implicit 'one word, therefore one thing' theory of language. Giorgi's account of 'jealousy' suggests that he is one of them. In this case, 'empathy' is a single word, so it must designate a single thing. Since the word is clearly used in a variety of ways, that must mean that there are several 'dimensions', 'components', or 'attributes' of empathy. The concept must be 'complex' and 'elusive', and defining it will be a difficult but necessary project. This theory of language is the starting point (or the hidden assumption) in many PQR studies. Thankfully, Batson does not appear to hold this view. Unfortunately, Tavakol *et al.* do hold it. Note two of their questions to the student respondents: 'Can you tell me how you see empathy in the context of patient care?' 'Can you tell me how empathy can be enhanced during medical education?' Both of these questions clearly imply that 'empathy' refers to just one thing.

17   Another way of looking at these findings is to say that, on average, students scored individual items on the JSPE(S) at 5.75 in the first three administrations, and at 5.45 in the fourth (at the end of Year 3). This does not look as if it merits the description 'cynicism develops progressively during their training' (Hojat *et al.* 2009: 1185), and leads one to wonder which items account for the six-point drop. Another study (Hojat *et al.* 2002) suggests that the mean JSPE score for 704 practising physicians is 120. So it may be that empathy levels recover – and then some – after graduation.

18   Or possibly state (viii), depending on how 'touched' is interpreted.

19   Additional ideas can, of course, be identified by following up references and Googling. There is, for instance, an interesting literature on the effects of nasally administered oxytocin on prosocial behaviour and empathic accuracy (through the recognition of facial expressions registering emotion). An example is Van Ijzendoorn and Bakermans-Kranenburg (2012). Such references indicate how accurate recognition of facial expressions can be evaluated and, as a bonus, introduce the reader to the literature on oxytocin and its effects on empathy, trust, and prosocial behaviour.

20   This is a variant of Pawson and Tilley's (1997) interviewing strategy, which presents the researcher's theory, usually framed in the form of a proposed mechanism, to knowledgeable respondents and invites them to comment on it.

What we are suggesting here is that the researcher/interviewer should play a much more active role in *teaching* the overall conceptual structure of the investigation to the subject. In practice this involves paying far more attention to 'explanatory passages', to 'sectional' and 'linking' narratives, to 'flow paths' and answer 'sequences', to 'repeated' and 'checking questions' ... The true test of data is whether they capture correctly those aspects of the subject's understanding which are relevant to the researcher's theory.

(167/164: their italics)

21 The literature on response to questionnaires shows that it is highly sensitive to changes in question wording and question order, and that subtle variations can affect the respondent's understanding of the questions she is asked. Cognitive approaches to survey methodology have proposed explanations of this response sensitivity, focusing particularly on cues available to the respondent. The cues determine what is relevant when answering a given question – which beliefs the respondent samples on that occasion – and largely account for response instability (Tourangeau *et al.* 2000). As a consequence, errors can be traced to psychological and communicative processes, and survey questions can be analysed in terms of the cognitive operations they are likely to evoke. Moreover, an understanding of the cognitive processes implicated in answering questions has made it possible, in many cases, to control and reduce response errors (Willis 2005). This literature is rarely acknowledged in qualitative research. Indeed, those who write on qualitative methods usually reject the cognitive approach, believing that it is 'inappropriate to see social interaction as "bias" which can potentially be eradicated' (Mason 2002: 65). This is to fly in the face of the evidence that people's response to questions varies considerably as a function of how those questions are asked. For a good explanation of why qualitative methods are especially prone to cognitive bias, see Trout (1998), Chapter 8.

22 Adams *et al.* (1999) is a review of self-report studies concerned with the extent to which clinicians adhere to guidelines. 'On average, clinicians tended to over-estimate their adherence to recommended norms by a median absolute difference of 27 per cent.' (190). The authors suggest that social desirability bias and interviewer bias probably account for this, adding: 'We would expect this form of bias to be greatest when the interviewer is a respected colleague or leader in the field'. Medical students interviewed by university educators about their adherence to ethical norms might find themselves in a similar position.

23 The problem with allowing respondents to 'use their own words' is that you are dependent on their vocabularies. If they don't express themselves very precisely, your attempt to 'describe the phenomenon on its own terms' is inevitably compromised by vagueness and ambiguity. For a topic like this, where the key term is intrinsically ambiguous, and there is a 'lack of consensus' about its meaning even in the literature, the findings will be (at best) very fuzzy.

24 A study by Marangoni *et al.* (1995) found that 'empathic accuracy in a clinical setting may require time to develop, regardless of the initial ability levels of the perceivers'. More specifically, it improves as a function of 'increased familiarity with the target individuals' (865), and is enhanced to an even greater extent if feedback is provided. So another bit of social psychology suggests that the sketch here might be on the right track, suggesting a mechanism that might account for the increasing cognitive ability of the students during Year 3.

25 Gross's (2002) discussion of emotion regulation could be used to refine the description of the two mechanisms referred to here: 'dialling down' and inhibition of expression. He discusses two methods of regulation:

The first, reappraisal, comes early in the emotion-generative process. It consists of changing the way a situation is construed so as to decrease its emotional impact.

The second, suppression, comes later in the emotion-generative process. It consists of inhibiting the outward signs of inner feelings.

(281)

It would appear that the medical students in Tavakol *et al.* adopted both types of regulation. Gross further notes that, according to a number of experimental studies, the reappraisal strategy is often more effective than suppression.

26   The classic work on these mechanisms was done by Asch (1955, 1961). However, his findings are often overstated and misinterpreted in textbooks. See Friend *et al.* (1990) and Jetten and Hornsey (2012). Still, it is not disputed that Asch's experiments recorded a sizeable minority of 'conformity' responses, even when this involved going along with what subjects perceived as an obviously incorrect judgment. However, it should be noted that there were marked individual differences, with only 5 per cent of participants *always* being swayed by the group.

References

6, P., and Bellamy, C. (2012) *Principles of Methodology: Research Design in Social Science.* London: Sage.

Adams, A. S., Soumerai, S. B., Lomas, J., and Ross-Degnan, D. (1999) 'Evidence of self-report bias in assessing adherence to guidelines', *International Journal for Quality in Health Care*, 11(3), pp. 187–192.

Asch, S. E. (1955) 'Opinions and social pressure', *Scientific American,* 193(5), pp. 31–35.

Asch, S. E. (1961) 'Effects of group pressure on modification and distortion of judgments', in M. Henle (ed.) *Documents of Gestalt Psychology.* Berkeley, CA: University of California Press, pp. 222–236.

Atsalos, C., Biggs, K., Boensch, S., Gavegan, F. L., Heath, S., Payk, M., and Trapolini, G. (2014) 'How clinical nurse and midwifery consultants optimise patient care in a tertiary referral hospital', *Journal of Clinical Nursing*, 23(19–20), pp. 2874–2885.

Bailer-Jones, D. (2008) 'Standing up against tradition: models and theories in Nancy Cartwright's Philosophy of Science', in S. Hartmann, C. Hoefer, and L. Bovens (eds.) *Nancy Cartwright's Philosophy of Science.* New York: Routledge, pp. 17–37.

Bailer-Jones, D. (2009) *Scientific Models in Philosophy of Science.* Pittsburgh, PA: University of Pittsburgh Press.

Batson, C. D. (2009) 'These things called empathy: eight related but distinct phenomena', in J. Decety, and W. Ickes (eds.) *The Social Neuroscience of Empathy.* Cambridge, MA: The MIT Press, pp. 3–15.

Batson, C.D. (2011) *Altruism in Humans.* New York: Oxford University Press.

Bechtel, W. (2007) *Mental Mechanisms: Philosophical Perspectives on Cognitive Neuroscience.* London: Routledge.

Bechtel, W., and Richardson, R. C. (2010) *Discovering Complexity: Decomposition and Localization as Strategies in Scientific Research.* Cambridge, MA: The MIT Press.

Bradbury-Jones, C., Irvine, F., and Sambrook, S. (2010) 'Empowerment of nursing students in clinical practice: spheres of influence', *Journal of Advanced Nursing*, 66(9), pp. 2061–2070.

Bruce, S. (2013) 'Post-secularity and religion in Britain: an empirical assessment', *Journal of Contemporary Religion*, 28(3), pp. 369–384.

Bryman, A. (2016) *Social Research Methods.* 5th edition. Oxford: Oxford University Press.

Carman, T. (2003) *Heidegger's Analytic: Interpretation, Discourse, and Authenticity in Being and Time.* Cambridge, UK: Cambridge University Press.

Chen, D., Lew, R., Hershman, W., and Orlander, J. A. (2007) 'A cross-sectional measurement of medical student empathy', *Journal of General Internal Medicine*, 22(10), pp. 1434–1438.

Cooper, J. L. (2007) *Cognitive Dissonance: 50 Years of Classic Theory.* London: Sage.

Craver, C. F. (2007) *Explaining the Brain.* Oxford: Oxford University Press.

Craver, C. F., and Darden, L. (2013) *In Search of Mechanisms: Discoveries Across the Life Sciences.* Chicago: University of Chicago Press.

Crotser, C. B., and Dickerson, S. S. (2010) 'Women receiving news of a family BRCA1/2 mutation: messages of fear and empowerment', *Journal of Nursing Scholarship*, 42(4), pp. 367–378.

Decety, J. (2014) *Empathy: From Bench to Bedside.* Cambridge, MA: The MIT Press.

Decety, J., and Ickes, W. (2009) *The Social Neuroscience of Empathy.* Cambridge, MA: The MIT Press.

Dovidio, J. F., Piliavin, J. A., Schoeder, D. A., and Penner, L. A. (2006) *The Social Psychology of Prosocial Behavior.* New York: Psychology Press.

Elmir, R., Jackson, D., Beale, B., and Schmied, V. (2010) 'Against all odds: Australian women's experiences of recovery from breast cancer', *Journal of Clinical Nursing*, 19(17–18), pp. 2531–2538.

Elster, J. (1983) *Explaining Technical Change: A Case Study in the Philosophy of Science.* Cambridge, UK: Cambridge University Press.

Elster, J. (2007) *Explaining Social Behaviour: More Nuts and Bolts for the Social Sciences.* Cambridge, UK: Cambridge University Press.

Festinger, L., and Carlsmith, J. M. (1959) 'Cognitive consequences of forced compliance', *Journal of Abnormal and Social Psychology*, 58(2), pp. 203–210.

Francis, R. (2013) *Report of the Mid Staffordshire NHS Foundation Trust Public Inquiry.* London: The Stationery Office.

Franck, R., and Iannaccone, L. R. (2014) 'Religious decline in the 20th century West: testing alternative explanations', *Public Choice*, 159(3), pp. 395–414.

Friend, R., Rafferty, Y., and Bramel, D. (1990) 'A puzzling misinterpretation of the Asch "conformity" study', *European Journal of Social Psychology*, 20(1), pp. 29–44.

Frigg, R., and Hartmann, S. (2012) 'Models in Science', in *Stanford Encyclopedia of Philosophy*, http://plato.stanford.edu/entries/models-science/. Retrieved 14th December 2015.

Frivold, G., Dale, B., and Slettebø, Â. (2015) 'Family members' experiences of being cared for by nurses and physicians in Norwegian intensive care units: a phenomenological hermeneutical study', *Intensive and Critical Care Nursing*, 31(4), pp. 232–240.

Gawronski, B. (2012) 'Back to the future of dissonance theory: cognitive consistency as a core motive', *Social Cognition*, 30(6), pp. 652–668.

Giere, R. N. (2006) *Scientific Perspectivism.* Chicago: University of Chicago Press.

Gladstein, G. A. (1983) 'Understanding empathy: integrating counselling, developmental, and social psychology perspectives', *Journal of Counseling Psychology*, 30(4), pp. 467–482.

Gross, J. J. (2002) 'Emotion regulation: affective, cognitive, and social consequences', *Psychophysiology*, 39(3), pp. 281–291.

Hacking, I. (2000) *The Social Construction of What?* Cambridge, MA: Harvard University Press.

Hamilton, W. D. (1967) 'Extraordinary sex ratios', *Science*, 156(3774), pp. 477–488.

Hartmann, S., Hoefer, C., and Bovens, L. (2008) *Nancy Cartwright's Philosophy of Science.* New York: Routledge.

Haynes, W. M. (2015) *CRC Handbook of Chemistry and Physics*. 96th edition. Boca Raton, FL: CRC Press.

Hedström, P., and Swedberg, R. (1998) *Social mechanisms: An Analytical Approach to Social Theory*. Cambridge, UK: Cambridge University Press.

Heidegger, M. (1962) *Being and Time*. Oxford: Basil Blackwell.

Hojat, M., Gonnella, J. S., Nasca, T., Mangione, S., Vergare, M. J., and Magee, J. C. (2002) 'Physician empathy: definition components, measurement, and relationship to gender and specialty', *The American Journal of Psychiatry*, 159(9), pp. 1563–1569.

Hojat, M., Gonnella, J. S., Mangione, S., Nasca, T., and Magee, J. C. (2003) 'Physician empathy in medical education and practice: experience with the Jefferson Scale of Physician Empathy', *Seminars in Integrative Medicine*, 1(1), pp. 25–41.

Hojat, M., Mangione, S., Nasca, T., Rattner, S., Erdmann, J. B., Gonnella, J. S., and Magee, J. C. (2004) 'An empirical study of decline in empathy in medical school', *Medical Education*, 38(9), pp. 934–941.

Hojat, M., Vergare, M. J., Maxwell, K., Brainard, G., Herrine, S. K., Isenberg, G. A., Veloski, J., and Gonnella, J. S. (2009) 'The devil is in the third year: a longitudinal study of erosion of empathy in medical school', *Academic Medicine*, 84(9), pp. 1182–1191.

Ickes, W. (2009) 'Empathic accuracy: its links to clinical, cognitive, developmental, social. and physiological psychology', in J. Decety, and W. Ickes (eds.) *The Social Neuroscience of Empathy*. Cambridge, MA: The MIT Press, pp. 57–70.

Jackson, J., and Morrissette, P. J. (2014) 'Exploring the experience of Canadian registered psychiatric nurses: a phenomenological study', *Journal of Psychiatric and Mental Health Nursing*, 21(2), pp. 138–144.

Jetten, J., and Hornsey, M. J. (2012) 'Conformity: revisiting Asch's line-judgment studies', in J. R. Smith, and S. A. Haslam (eds.) *Social Psychology: Revisiting the Classic Studies*. Los Angeles: Sage, pp. 76–90.

LaPorte, J. (2004) *Natural Kinds and Conceptual Change*. Cambridge, UK: Cambridge University Press.

Lee, H. Y., Hsu, M.-T., Li, P.-L., and Sloan, R. S. (2013) ' "Struggling to be an insider": a phenomenological design of new nurses' transition', *Journal of Clinical Nursing*, 22(5–6), pp. 789–797.

Marangoni, C., Garcia, S., Ickes, W., and Teng, G. (1995) 'Empathic accuracy in a clinically relevant setting', *Journal of Personality and Social Psychology*, 68(5), pp. 854–869.

Mason, J. (2002) *Qualitative Researching*. 2nd edition. London: Sage.

Mayo, D. G. (1996) *Error and the Growth of Experimental Knowledge*. Chicago: University of Chicago Press.

Miles, M., and Huberman, A. (1994) *Qualitative Data Analysis*. London: Sage.

Morgan, M. S., and Morrison, M. (eds.) (1999) *Models as Mediators: Perspectives on Natural and Social Science*. Cambridge, UK: Cambridge University Press.

Morrison, M., and Morgan, M.S. (1999) 'Models as mediating instruments', in M. S. Morgan, and M. Morrison (eds.) *Models as Mediators: Perspectives on Natural and Social Science*. Cambridge, UK: Cambridge University Press, pp. 10–37.

Moses, J.W., and Knutsen, T.L. (2012) *Ways of Knowing: Competing Methodologies in Social and Political Research*. Basingstoke, UK: Palgrave Macmillan.

Newton, B. W., Barber, I., Clardy, J., and Cleveland, E. (2008) 'Is there hardening of the heart during medical school?', *Academic Medicine*, 83(3), pp. 244–249.

Paley, J. (2005) 'Phenomenology as rhetoric', *Nursing Inquiry*, 12(2), pp. 106–116.

Paley, J. (2014a) 'Heidegger, lived experience and method', *Journal of Advanced Nursing*, 70(7), pp. 1520–1531.

Paley, J. (2014b) 'Cognition and the compassion deficit: the social psychology of helping behaviour in nursing', *Nursing Philosophy*, 15(4), pp. 274–287.

Pawson, R., and Tilley, N. (1997) *Realistic Evaluation.* London: Sage.

Rosenthal, S., Howard, B., Schlussel, Y., Herrigal, D., Smolarz, B. G., Gable, B., Vasquez, J., Grigo, H., and Kaufman, M. (2011) 'Humanism at heart: preserving empathy in third-year medical students', *Academic Medicine*, 86(3), pp. 350–358.

Sherman, J. J., and Cramer, A. (2005) 'A measurement of changes in empathy during dental school', *Journal of Dental Education*, 69(3), pp. 338–345.

Sherwood, H. (2016) 'Church of England weekly attendance falls below 1m for the first time' *Guardian*, 12 January 2016. Available at: www.theguardian.com/world/2016/jan/2012/church-of-england-attendance-falls-below-million-first-time.

Silverman, D. (2000) *Doing Qualitative Research: A Practical Handbook.* London: Sage.

Smith, J. (2007) 'Hermeneutics, human sciences and health: linking theory and practice', *International Journal of Qualitative Studies on Health and Well-being*, 2(1), pp. 3–11.

Spiro, H. (2009) 'Commentary: the practice of empathy', *Academic Medicine*, 84(9), pp. 1177–1179.

Tavakol, S., Dennick, R., and Tavakol, M. (2012) 'Medical students' understanding of empathy: a phenomenological study', *Medical Education*, 46(3), pp. 306–316.

Thorkildsen, K., and Råholm, M.-B. (2010) 'The essence of professional competence experienced by Norwegian nurse students: a phenomenological study', *Nurse Education in Practice*, 10(4), pp. 183–188.

Thurang, A., Fagerberg, I., Palmstierna, T., and Tops, A. B. (2010) 'Women's experiences of caring when in treatment for alcohol dependency', *Scandinavian Journal of Caring Sciences*, 24(4), pp. 700–706.

Tourangeau, R., Rips, I. J., and Rasinski, K. (2000) *The Psychology of Survey Response.* Cambridge, UK: Cambridge University Press.

Trout, J.D. (1998) *Measuring the Intentional World: Realism, Naturalism, and Quantitative Methods in the Behavioral Sciences.* New York: Oxford University Press.

van Dijk, T.A. (1996) 'Discourse, power and access', in C. R. Caldas-Coulthard, and C. Coulthard (eds.) *Texts and Practices: Readings in Critical Discourse Analysis.* London: Routledge, pp. 84–106.

Van Ijzendoorn, M. H., and Bakermans-Kranenburg, M. J. (2012) 'A sniff of trust: meta-analysis of the effects of intranasal oxytocin administration on face recognition, trust to in-group, and trust to out-group', *Psychoneuroendocrinology*, 37(3), pp. 438–443.

Weisberg, M. (2013) *Simulation and Similarity: Using Models to Understand the World.* Oxford: Oxford University Press.

Widdowson, H. G. (2004) *Text, Context, Pretext: Critical Issues in Discourse Analysis.* Oxford: Blackwell Publishing.

Willis, G. B. (2005) *Cognitive Interviewing: A Tool for Improving Questionnaire Design.* Thousand Oaks, CA: Sage.

Wittenbrink, B., and Schwarz, N. (2007) *Implicit Measures of Attitudes.* New York: Guilford Press.

Wyatt, T. (2014) 'C of E attendance statistics slope still points downwards', *Church Times*, 14 November 2014. Available at: www.churchtimes.co.uk/articles/2014/2014-november/news/uk/c-of-e-attendance-statistics-slope-still-points-downward. Retrieved 2011/2012/2015.

Index

Page numbers in *italics* denote tables, those in **bold** denote figures.

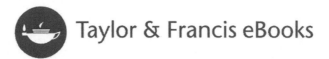

Printed and bound by CPI Group (UK) Ltd, Croydon, CR0 4YY

17/10/2024

01775686-0013